COMING OUT

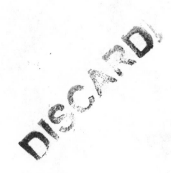

EMPOWERING YOU

The Rowman & Littlefield Empowering You series is aimed to help you, as a young adult, deal with important topics that you, your friends, or family might be facing. Whether you are looking for answers about certain illnesses, social issues, or personal problems, the books in this series provide you with the most up-to-date information. Throughout each book you will also find stories from other teenagers to provide personal perspectives on the subject.

COMING OUT

Insights and Tips for Teenagers

KEZIA ENDSLEY

ROWMAN & LITTLEFIELD
Lanham • Boulder • New York • London

Published by Rowman & Littlefield
An imprint of The Rowman & Littlefield Publishing Group, Inc.
4501 Forbes Boulevard, Suite 200, Lanham, Maryland 20706
www.rowman.com

6 Tinworth Street, London, SE11 5AL, United Kingdom

British Library Cataloguing in Publication Information Available

Library of Congress Cataloging-in-Publication Data

Names: Endsley, Kezia, 1968– author.
Title: Coming out : insights and tips for teenagers / Kezia Endsley.
Description: Lanham : Rowman & Littlefield, 2020. | Series: Empowering you | Includes bibliographical references and index. | Audience: Grades 10–12 | Summary: "This book addresses the hows and whys of coming out, as well as potential concerns teenagers may have—including how to know when you're ready to come out, who to tell first, and how to deal with unsupportive people. Firsthand accounts from teenagers provide personal insight throughout"— Provided by publisher.
Identifiers: LCCN 2020029326 (print) | LCCN 2020029327 (ebook) | ISBN 9781538135730 (paperback) | ISBN 9781538135747 (ebook)
Subjects: LCSH: Coming out (Sexual orientation)—Juvenile literature. | Teenagers—Sexual behavior—Juvenile literature.
Classification: LCC HQ76.26.E553 2020 (print) | LCC HQ76.26 (ebook) | DDC 306.76/6—dc23
LC record available at https://lccn.loc.gov/2020029326
LC ebook record available at https://lccn.loc.gov/2020029327

CONTENTS

YOU ARE NOT ALONE

I think being gay is a blessing, and it's
something I am thankful for every single day.
—Anderson Cooper, American journalist,
television personality, and author

SEEKING A BETTER UNDERSTANDING

If you are picking up this book, you are likely wondering if you fall somewhere on the LGBTQIA+ spectrum. Beyond just feeling "different," maybe you have begun to wonder if you might be gay (or lesbian, queer, bisexual, or trans) or some other label you prefer. Many people have mixed feelings when they first try on a new way of identifying. It can be a mix of excitement, relief, and worry. Maybe you know exactly who you are but are afraid or don't know how to tell the people in your life. In any case, this book can help.

Revealing your homosexuality is never easy—no matter your age—but the process can be particularly challenging for teens, who still depend on their families financially, emotionally, and otherwise. You have probably not yet established your own private life with your own place to live and a job to provide financial support. The fact is, suicide is the second leading cause of death among all young people ages ten to twenty-four,[1] and LGBTQIA+ youth seriously contemplate suicide at almost three times the rate of heterosexual youth.[2] This fact is mainly because they can't see a way past the rejection from their families and other loved ones.

The news isn't all doom and gloom, however. The Human Rights Campaign's 2012 report, entitled "Growing Up LGBT in America," reported the following heartening trends:

- Nine out of ten LGBTQ+ youth said that they are out to their close friends.

- Sixty-four percent reported that they were out to their classmates.

- Seventy-five percent reported that most of their peers did not have a problem with their identity as LGBTQ+.

- More than three-quarters (77 percent) of LGBTQ+ youth reported that they know things will get better.[3]

The report, in general, found these youth to be extraordinarily resilient. LGBTQ+ teens find safe havens among their peers, online, and in their schools. They generally remain optimistic and believe things will get better.[4]

Those feelings seem to be grounded in facts and figures, too. For example, a survey by Pew Research Center in 2017, found that 63 percent of Americans said in 2016, that homosexuality should be accepted by society,[5] compared with 51 percent in 2006. LGBTQ+ adults recognize the change in attitudes: In another survey by Pew Research Center in 2013, of adults identifying as LGBTQIA+, about nine in ten (92 percent) said that society had become more accepting of them in the previous decade.[6] As you may know, in 2015, the U.S. Supreme Court struck down all state bans on gay marriage and legalized it in all fifty states. A 2019 Gallup Poll reported that 73 percent of those polled agreed that gay marriage should be legal.[7]

Regardless of the changing attitudes in the broader United States or your hometown, only you can decide when and how you come out. You may have realized that living your truth without fear of being "found out" would be a liberating, self-affirming, and powerful thing to do. Yet, it's much easier said than done. This book cannot promise that your family and friends will unconditionally accept you, but it can prepare you for the various responses you might get and help you deal with them honestly and openly.

HENRY'S STORY

Henry was fifteen when he decided he could not keep his secret any longer. He had known he was gay for almost ten years at that point. Okay, maybe he didn't exactly know the word "gay" at five, but he knew he was wired a certain way, and it became obvious to him later what that meant. He grew up in a religious, conservative area of the country with devout parents, so coming out wasn't a decision he took lightly. Henry was starting to have real crushes on boys he knew (rather than celebs and YouTube stars), and he wanted his family to know before he started dating anyone.

One Sunday, he came home from church after his conservative pastor had given his most homophobic sermon yet. He felt so unvalued and "wrong," and he went into his bedroom and sobbed. His mom heard him and asked why he was crying. But the words were too difficult to speak. She put things together and realized that he was upset about the sermon. She finally asked, "Do you think you're gay?" That's when Henry told her. The first thing she said is that she would always love him. They talked for an hour. He cried the entire time, but they were tears of relief.

Even though the initial coming out was better than Henry had feared, his parents had to take the long journey of reconciling their religious beliefs with their love for Henry. The first year was particularly hard, and he fought a lot with them. Throughout time, the yelling turned into conversations and, eventually, understanding. His parents eventually met his boyfriend at the time and began asking him questions about his dating life. They were able to find common ground, despite their different beliefs.

Henry stresses that coming out is not a one-time proclamation. It's a process that takes patience and understanding from both ends. Even though it took work and time to find peace with his family, he says that coming out felt like the biggest weight that ever came off his shoulders.

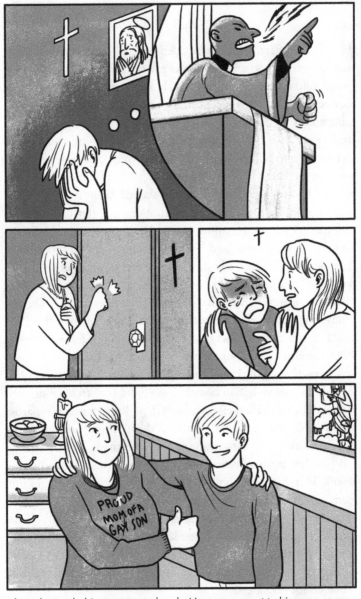

After a homophobic sermon at church, Henry came out to his mom as gay, and together they worked through reconciling their beliefs. *Illustration by Kate Haberer*

LGBTQIA+ AND BEYOND:
WHAT DOES IT ALL MEAN?

What does LGBTQIA+ stand for? Let's break it down. The letters represent, in order, lesbian, gay, bisexual, transgender, questioning (or queer), intersex, and ally (or asexual). The plus means anyone else who was inadvertently not included. Some people prefer LGBT, some use LGBTQ, and some even use QILTBAG (that's just LGBTQIA in an order that makes a word of sorts). There is no one correct way, and this ever-expanding acronym is one of the reasons some people prefer to use "queer" as an umbrella term.

There are many different ways that people understand and identify themselves. Sexuality and gender are just two of those many ways. As the world becomes more open and accepting, sexuality and gender are both more commonly viewed as fluid.

Instead of attempting (and most likely failing) to include all the identity categories in this book, the focus is on teens questioning their sexuality. To try to cover teens questioning their sexuality and teens questioning their gender identity in such a short book would inevitably give short shrift to both issues. You'll read much more about sexual identity in chapter 1. For resources on gender identity, see the "Resources" section at the end of this book.

WHAT DOES IT MEAN TO COME OUT?

Coming out starts with facing your truth yourself—essentially coming out to yourself. Where do you fall in the LGBTQIA+ spectrum? Is your concept of your sexuality and gender free-flowing, or is it consistent? Maybe you don't know what to "call" yourself yet. That's okay, too. Questioning is a normal and healthy part of growing up.

It's also normal to wonder about coming out. On the one hand, it might feel like a relief. Friends might be asking questions that you avoid or struggle to answer. Finally, you can be honest. On the other hand, you probably think about how your world could change: How will people react? Will the people you tell spread the word to someone you'd prefer not to know?

Most people come out gradually. They start by telling a counselor or a few close friends or family. A lot of people tell a counselor or therapist because they want to be sure their information remains private. Some call a LGBTQIA+ support group so they can have help working through their feelings about identity or coming out.

AT WHAT AGE DOES A PERSON KNOW?

According to a 2013 Pew Research Center poll—a lesbian, gay, and bisexual survey—respondents were asked how old they were when they first felt they might be something other than straight or heterosexual. The median age across all LGBTQIA+ adults is twelve. On average, gay men reported thinking at about age ten that they might not be straight. For both lesbians and bisexuals, the median age was thirteen.[8]

Another good first step for many teens is to reach out to other LGBTQIA+ teens. If you are fortunate enough to know some or know of supportive groups, this can be a positive first step. If you don't know any people in your hometown, you can find many like-minded and supportive groups online. As you begin feeling more comfortable with your identity, you can begin to come out to others. Many teens come out to one or another parent first, some to both at the same time. Everyone's journey is different.

Don't pressure yourself about the process of coming out by creating an artificial deadline. Depending on your circumstances, the coming-out process may take you six months, five years, ten years, or a lifetime. Coming out is a process of self-discovery, and each person has their own personal journey, timetable, and destination.

USE OF THE WORD QUEER

Although the word "queer" has been used in the past to refer to gay people pejoratively, it's becoming an increasingly accepted term within the LGBTQIA+ community, especially with younger people. Language evolves, and this word has been "taken back" by many in the LGBTQIA+ community as a word of pride. The reason it's used sometimes in this book is to honor the choice of many LGBTQIA+ youth.

DEALING WITH SELF-LOATHING AND BUILDING SELF-RESPECT

A common theme throughout this book is how you can build your self-esteem and self-respect, and learn to love and accept yourself, just the way you are. It's hard to be a teenager—and even harder when you are questioning or queer. Coming to terms with this and learning to love yourself—despite the many messages you may get from your family, your school, your church, the media, etc.—takes work.

I believe that you have to accept yourself first before you can bring anyone who's struggling [with acceptance] along with you.
—Eric, identifies as gay, age eighteen

It's a journey but one well worth taking. Remember that you are not alone. This book and the references therein can help guide you in finding the connections and support you need to be the best "you" you can be. It does get better. With time, you will see that your differences become a source of pride and strength. Your struggles will give you compassion and wisdom. Chapter 2 covers this journey in more detail.

xiv   YOU ARE NOT ALONE

> The National Suicide Prevention Lifeline number is 1-800-273-8255. Reach out for help. Things will get better!

FINDING SUPPORTIVE PEER GROUPS

As part of coming out or even before you begin talking to peers, family, or friends, it will help your process immensely if you can find like-minded and accepting peers, counselors, teachers, or friends who can lend you support and advice.

IT GETS BETTER

Check out the "It Gets Better" project, at itgetsbetter.org or on YouTube at www.youtube.com/user/itgetsbetterproject, created by journalist Dan Savage and his husband, Terry Miller. You can watch an endless stream of inspiring stories shared by LGBTQIA+ adults or use their "Get Help" page to find LGBTQIA+ youth support services in your area.

You can start finding online safe havens by checking out the Centers for Disease Control and Prevention's information site on LGBT youth resources at www.cdc.gov/lgbthealth/youth-resources.htm. Chapters 5 and 7 cover how to build a supportive friend group in more detail.

WHAT DOES THIS BOOK COVER?

This book addresses the hows and whys of coming out, as well as potential concerns you may have—from how to know when you're ready to come out to your community, to who to tell first, to how to deal with unsupportive people, and to how to move into loving self-acceptance.

Part I starts with a broad overview of recognizing your sexuality. It also offers encouragement and includes quotes and stories from teens who have had experience coming out. It provides guidelines, questions, and recommendations for helping you determine the best way to handle coming out, and how to handle it if someone "outs" you before you're ready. Here's a breakdown of the chapters in this part:

- Chapter 1 talks about the road to understanding your sexuality and personal identity.

- Chapter 2 talks about how to deal with negative feelings and build up your self-esteem.

- Chapter 3 talks about how and when to come out.

Part II addresses your expectations about each phase of the coming-out process. With quotes from teens who have already come out, this section highlights what they hoped to get from the experience, how or if those expectations were met, the challenges they faced along the way, and what surprised them most about their experiences.

This section also covers some questions you should be prepared to answer as you come out to people you care about, as well as dealing with family and friends who aren't supportive, keeping the dialogue open with family members who are struggling with acceptance, handling bullies, building a "support family" of accepting friends, and more. It also highlights the challenges teens face living out in today's world. One important issue you'll read about is how to deal with homophobia in a way that's healthy and affirming of who you are. The following is a breakdown of the chapters in this part:

- Chapter 4 discusses how to deal with reactions of all types.

- Chapter 5 discusses how to build a supportive network of friends, both locally and online.

Part III is all about living a fulfilling life as a gay person. It covers finding your "tribe" of friends and supporters, bringing home gay friends to meet your family, staying safe online, dealing with first dates and breakups, having a safe yet fulfilling sex life, and finding overall personal acceptance and love during your journey. Here's a breakdown of the chapters in this part:

- Chapter 6 talks about building safe, loving, and affirming sexual relationships.

- Chapter 7 details how you can live a fulfilling life when you're out and proud.

Good luck on your journey. We hope this book can help you along the way.

PART I

WHAT DOES COMING OUT REALLY MEAN?

CHAPTER ONE

UNDERSTANDING YOUR SEXUALITY AND PERSONAL IDENTITY

*When all Americans are treated as equal, no matter
who they are or whom they love, we are all more free.*
—Barack Obama, forty-fourth president of the United States

SEEKING A BETTER UNDERSTANDING

Our culture seems to be slowly realizing that sexual preference is on a spectrum, rather than being a binary (yes or no) kind of characteristic. Teen boys find themselves wanting another man, and teen girls find themselves wanting another woman. Some teens find that they are equally attracted to men and women, or sometimes to men and other times to women. All of this is normal.

If you're wondering if you're queer, the good news is you don't have to know the answer right now. Some feelings get stronger throughout time, and some get weaker. Since no two people experience desire and love in the same way, you can't just open a textbook that will teach you exactly who you are and what to do. This chapter hopes to help you along the path of self-exploration.

THE DIFFERENCE BETWEEN GENDER IDENTITY AND SEXUAL ORIENTATION

Whereas sexual orientation is considered an inherent and (usually) enduring emotional, romantic, or sexual attraction to other people, gender identity is a person's internal concept of self as male, female, a blend of both, or neither.[1] It's how individuals perceive themselves and what they call themselves. Your gender identity can be the same or different from your sex assigned at birth. Transgender people may be straight, lesbian, gay, or bisexual, just as cisgender people may be.

WHAT SHOULD I CALL YOU?

As a point of reference, the following tables (see tables 1.1 and 1.2) outline the various ways humans currently identify sexually and gender-wise. Of course, these terms and identities are fluid, and by the time you read this, there might changes. For the latest terminology, check out the Human Rights Campaign's site at www.hrc.org (try www .hrc.org/resources/glossary-of-terms, for example).

Table 1.1.   Sexual Identities and Their Definitions

Identity	Definition
gay	A person (male or female) who is emotionally, romantically, or sexually attracted to members of the same gender. Sometimes still refers to just men, as in "gay men and lesbians."
lesbian	A woman who is emotionally, romantically, or sexually attracted to other women.
bisexual	A person emotionally, romantically, or sexually attracted to more than one sex, gender, or gender identity, although not necessarily simultaneously, in the same way or to the same degree.
queer	A (once-derogatory) term people often use to express fluid identities and orientations. Often used interchangeably with LGBTQ.
pansexual	Someone who has the potential for emotional, romantic, or sexual attraction to people of any gender, although not necessarily simultaneously, in the same way or to the same degree.
asexual	Someone who experiences little to no sexual attraction.

Identity	Definition
demisexual	Someone who generally does not experience sexual attraction unless they have formed a strong emotional connection with someone.
graysexual	Someone who occasionally experiences sexual attraction but usually does not; it covers a kind of gray area between asexuality and sexual identity.

Sources: Human Rights Campaign, "Glossary of Terms," last modified 2020, https://www.hrc.org/resources/glossary-of-terms; Michael Gold, "The ABCs of L.G.B.T.Q.I.A.+," *New York Times*, last modified June 7, 2019, https://www.nytimes.com/2018/06/21/style/lgbtq-gender-language.html.

Table 1.2. Gender Identities and Their Definitions

Identity	Definition
transgender	Someone whose gender identity or expression is different from the biological sex they were assigned at birth.
transfeminine	An umbrella term used to describe someone who was assigned male at birth and identifies with femininity. Someone who identifies as transfeminine may also identify as a trans woman or female.
transmasculine	Someone who was assigned female at birth but identifies with masculinity. Someone who identifies as transmasculine may also identify as a trans man, trans woman, or male.
cisgender	Someone whose gender identity matches the sex they were assigned at birth.
genderqueer	Someone whose gender identity is outside the strict male and female binary. They may express both traditionally masculine and feminine qualities or neither.
gender nonconforming	Someone who expresses gender outside traditional norms associated with masculinity or femininity. Not all gender-nonconforming people are transgender, and some transgender people express gender in conventionally masculine or feminine ways.
nonbinary	Another term for someone who identifies as neither male nor female and sees themselves outside the gender binary (male and female as one of two choices only).
gender fluid	Someone whose identity shifts or fluctuates. These individuals may identify or express themselves as more masculine on some days and more feminine on others.
gender-neutral	Someone who prefers not to be described by a specific gender but prefers "they" as a singular pronoun or the "Mx.," a substitute for "Mr." or "Ms."
intersex	Someone who is born with reproductive or sexual anatomy that doesn't fit the typical definitions of female or male.
agender	Those who don't identify with any gender or can't relate to gender terms or labels at all. Agender people are not necessarily asexual. They can have any sexual orientation.

Sources: Human Rights Campaign, "Glossary of Terms," last modified 2020, https://www.hrc.org/resources/glossary-of-terms; Michael Gold, "The ABCs of L.G.B.T.Q.I.A.+," *New York Times*, last modified June 7, 2019, https://www.nytimes.com/2018/06/21/style/lgbtq-gender-language.html.

You might decide that you don't exactly fit into any of these categories, and that's okay, too. The important thing right now is to relax and start telling yourself, "Whatever the answer, it's my business; it's only part of who I am, and I'm going to grow to embrace it and like it about myself."

You can't let other people determine who you are attracted to—it'll just add misery to your life that you don't need. Be intentional. Listen to your body, mind, and heart.

MYTHS ABOUT SEXUAL ORIENTATION

Let's start by laying to rest some common myths about sexual orientation. You may have heard others say these things, or perhaps you've thought them yourself. It's time to dash these misconceptions to the rocks.

- *A person is either straight or gay.* When it comes to sexual orientation, many (most?) people are neither 100 percent straight nor 100 percent gay. Recent research indicates that, when given the option, many heterosexual people describe themselves as "mostly straight" rather than "straight."[2]

- *Everyone who claims to be bisexual is in denial about being gay.* See the text box titled "A Myth about Bisexuality" in this chapter.

- *A bisexual person is always equally attracted to both men and women.* Although some bisexuals feel equal or almost equal emotional and physical attractions to males and females, this is more often not the case. Bisexuals can be heterosexual-leaning, homosexual-leaning, or varied (have greater emotional attraction to one sex and greater physical attraction to the other sex).

- *A person's emotional and physical attractions should be the same.* Romantic love and sexual desire are fundamentally separate experiences that evolved for different reasons. There is no biological requirement that romantic love and sexual desire be congruent.[3]

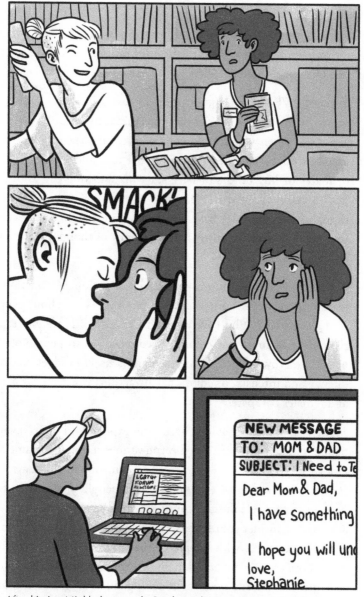

After kissing Mickhela at work, Stephanie began to accept that she was a lesbian and decided to come out to her parents through an e-mail.
Illustration by Kate Haberer

GATHERING THE EVIDENCE

Of course, thoughts, emotions, and behaviors are connected. For the sake of simplicity, however, you might want to try to identify evidence for each of these separately:

- *Thoughts:* What thoughts, including fantasies, have you had about others of the same sex? Your thoughts might include, "Wow, they are cute!" when you see someone of the same sex pass by. Your fantasies might include imagining what it would be like to date or marry or hug or kiss or have sex with someone you know, or with a celebrity, who is the same sex as you. Conversely, what thoughts and fantasies have you had about people of the other sex? How does the intensity and frequency of thoughts for males and females compare?

- *Emotions:* What emotions—especially emotional attraction— have you felt toward others of the same sex? What about people of the other sex? Who have you had a crush on? Have you experienced weak or absent emotional connections to people of the other sex? Toward people of the same sex? How does the frequency and intensity of emotional attractions you have for males and females compare?

- *Behaviors:* What behaviors have you experienced that involve people of the same sex? Maybe you've masturbated to same-sex erotica or your fantasies that involved someone of the same sex. If you have had sexual experiences with people of the same sex, how satisfying were those encounters, emotionally, as well as sexually? Also, consider your heterosexual experiences. If you have had sexual experiences with people of the other sex, how satisfying were those encounters emotionally, as well as sexually? Behaviors also include various types of touching, including hugging and kissing. What has been your response to experiences of touch with males and females?

CHAPTER TWO

DEALING WITH NEGATIVE FEELINGS AND BUILDING SELF-RESPECT

It takes some intelligence and insight to figure out you're gay and then a tremendous amount of balls to live it and live it proudly.
—Jason Bateman, actor and producer

SEEKING A BETTER UNDERSTANDING

Part of every person's process of maturing and growing up is accepting and ultimately loving who they are. The process is hard for all of us and can be especially challenging during the teen years. When you add being different in some way, the path is even more difficult. Additionally, you hear negative messages from your loved ones, the media, your religious community, and so on. It's no wonder that LGBTQIA+ teens report higher amounts of stress and depression, and greater thoughts of suicide on average, than non-LGBTQIA+ teens.[1] We live in a culture that wrongly assumes that being straight is better than being gay.

This chapter will help you come to terms with the impact on your self-esteem by the negative messages you've taken in about LGBTQIA+ people. It discusses methods you can use to modify that negative self-talk and heal. Healing and improving your self-esteem doesn't happen overnight. It's a lifelong process for most of us; however, the hard work is worth it.

Find out who you are and be that person. That's what your
soul was put on this Earth to be. Find that truth,
live that truth, and everything else will come.
—Ellen DeGeneres

Here are just some of the benefits of having a positive self-esteem/self-image:

- You'll feel confident in asserting your needs and opinions.

- You'll build strong convictions but also be more open to new evidence.

- You'll be willing to accept responsibility, as appropriate.

- You'll have an optimistic attitude.

- You'll have more secure, strong, and honest relationships.

- You'll feel more self-motivated.

- You'll have realistic expectations and be less critical of yourself and others.

- Your overall performance and risk-taking ability will improve.

WHAT HAS INFLUENCED YOUR SELF-ESTEEM?

Self-esteem is essentially confidence or an overall feeling of self-worth and value that a person has about themselves. Most psychologists feel that we are all born with healthy self-esteem, which is then either nurtured or damaged by our life experiences. If you suffer from low self-esteem (or self-worth), a good first step to feeling better is to look at the factors that have led to your feeling this way.

Risk factors for LGBTQIA+ people include negative experiences (e.g., discrimination, victimization), negative attitudes toward homosexuality, your internal discomfort with sexual identity, and your emotional suffering related to acceptance.

and anxiety while having little or no potential for achieving changes in orientation.[12]

Perhaps because of these findings and support, as of 2020, nineteen states, the District of Columbia, and Puerto Rico have passed laws protecting LGBTQIA+ youth from conversion therapy by licensed practitioners. These states include California, New Jersey, Illinois, Oregon, Vermont, Connecticut, Nevada, New Mexico, Rhode Island, Washington State, New York, Maryland, Hawaii, New Hampshire, Massachusetts, Colorado, Maine, Maryland, and Utah. Many cities and municipalities have bans on conversion therapy for minors, for instance, Cincinnati, Ohio, and West Palm Beach, Florida.

The conversion methods are based on intolerant, inaccurate, and outdated assumptions about gender and sexual orientation. Moreover, they don't work. There is nothing wrong with your sexual orientation. You don't need to be fixed because you are not broken.

MESSAGES FROM PEERS AND SCHOOL

Social pressures are part of the school experience of many students, regardless of sexual orientation or gender identity. They can be particularly difficult for LGBTQIA+ students, who often struggle to make sense of their identities, don't have support from family and friends, and continuously hear negative messaging about LGBTQIA+ people at school and in their communities. It is estimated that LGBTQIA+ young people are three times as likely as their peers to drop out of high school (often because they feel unsafe and suffer abuse), and many who drop out do not get a GED, let alone go on to college.[13]

You've likely heard slurs and put-downs at school, and maybe even experienced some violence because you're "different" and watched as teachers sat by and did nothing. If so, you are a typical LGBTQIA+ teen. The messages you hear from peers are echoes of the culture they live in—the same homophobic culture in which we all exist.

The most hurtful of these can be "casual" comments made by friends. It sometimes helps to remember that these comments are made out of ignorance, and the antidote to ignorance is education. Of course, it's not your job to educate your peers about hate and ignorance, but if it gives you feelings of pride and self-worth to do so, then good for you.

One way to combat such abuse is to organize a Gay–Straight Alliance (GSA) at your school. Such a club can provide essential resources for students and give you and others supportive spaces to counteract bullying and institutional silence about issues of importance to you. Not every school is open to such clubs, however. Sometimes, your best course of action is to stay in the closet until you have a safe place to come out. Just because your peers can't accept you at this time doesn't mean you can't begin the process of healing.

THE JOURNEY OF HEALING

The goal here is to reject the attitudes, behaviors, and beliefs that aren't working for you and, more importantly, start to identify and develop ones that are. The first step is to bring these attitudes and behaviors to awareness, where they can be compassionately examined and then left behind, resulting in a much happier life.

PROFESSIONAL HELP

For professional help with your journey, there are lots of places you can turn. The Trevor Project (www.thetrevorproject.org) has a crisis intervention LifeLine (1-866-488-7386); TrevorChat for confidential online instant messaging with a Trevor counselor; TrevorText (text START to 678678) for confidential online text messaging with a Trevor counselor; and TrevorSpace (www.trevor space.org), an online international peer-to-peer community for LGBTQIA+ young people and their friends. You can also go online for therapy at www.talkspace.com/online-therapy/lgbtq/. To find a counselor in your area who specializes in LGBTQIA+ issues, visit www.pridecounseling.com.

You may find truth in these simple words: No one can label you but you. It sounds straightforward, but there is a lot of power in claiming your identity, and it positively affects your emotional health. Accepting and loving your identity isn't easy, but it's worth it.

FEEL THE FEELINGS

The first step is coming to know more about your pain. It can seem counterintuitive to lean into the pain, but you have to understand the problem before you can work on it effectively.

Suffering is universal; in fact, that is a central principle of Buddhist teachings. Fear can keep us from looking at the actual root of a problem. If we allow ourselves to search for the origin of our suffering, we can then begin to face it.

You can explore and face your suffering through meditation, art, mindfulness, therapy, or another way. It won't be easy, but chances are when you realize the depth and extent of your suffering, you will also recognize the hope, possibility, and growth opportunity.

MODIFY NEGATIVE SELF-TALK

Automatic thoughts are typically the easiest to see and begin to address. One way to go about this is to keep track of your automatic thoughts as they happen. Write them down. After you have tracked them for a while (say, one week), take some time to go back through them and look for patterns. The regularly recurring thoughts can give you insight into the core beliefs you hold about yourself. Once you recognize some of the patterns, think about the emotional costs of these thoughts and beliefs. Are they benefitting you? Are they even true?

You can then begin the process of replacing negative beliefs with more healthy, accurate, and effective self-statements. You will then start feeling the positive changes in your self-esteem. Table 2.1 shows the emotional costs of negative thoughts and suggests healthy thoughts as replacements.

The next step is to recognize and challenge your old ways of thinking. Evaluate the effectiveness, usefulness, and bias of these thoughts.

Table 2.1.   The Emotional Cost of Negative Thoughts

Thought Pattern	Emotional Cost	Healthy Thought
I'm bad. I'm weird.	I feel less than and separate from others, and otherwise just unworthy.	There are many people just like me in the world. The LGBTQIA+ community is large and thriving, even if I don't see it where I am right now.
Other people are happier and more together than I am.	I feel at fault for being unhappy and less than for not managing better.	Most people put on a mask when in public. I am struggling with my identity, and that's hard, so I have a right to be confused and unhappy right now.
I am/will be a huge disappointment to my family (when I come out).	I feel that I will never be loved as I am.	I am lovable, just the way I am. I will find a loving community.

This battle is more difficult when you continue to hear distorted and negative messages daily. Every time you are bullied at school, hear a homophobic joke, listen to a story about gay-bashing, or watch a heterocentric advertisement, you receive direct and indirect messages that suggest you are inferior, damaged, or worthless.

TREAT YOURSELF KINDLY

If you struggle with treating yourself kindly, try this mental exercise. Imagine you have a younger sister or brother, several years younger than you, who you love dearly and is struggling with things you remember struggling with at that age. If your kind words and actions could help that younger person, what would you do and say? Now imagine that the person is your younger self. Your younger self is just a child who doesn't understand all the reasons why they suffer. So many things that happen to them are out of their control. Can you show that same compassion and kindness toward them? Finally, how about showing compassion to the present-day you? Imagine the thirty-year-old you, who is wiser and more comfortable in their skin. How would that person comfort and help you today, if they could?

Your special challenge is to overcome the negative messages from your family of origin and childhood, and actively challenge negative messages in the media and your community. It sounds like a lot of work, but throughout time, you will become skilled at recognizing distortions or biases that are held as "universal truths." The messages will still be out there, but you will no longer "let them in." You will have the ability to see them as they are and not let them define you or damage your self-esteem any longer.

LET GO OF SHAME

Shame is an outward feeling, in the sense that we feel it in relation to how the world sees us. It's like humiliation—a bad feeling because of how we look to others. We can feel guilt inwardly, without an audience, but we need others to feel shame. Core shame usually indicates early psychological damage that can hinder your growth to adulthood. For LGBTQIA+ people, shame can be a significant barrier to happiness.

Darrell C. Greene, a psychologist in private practice in New York, looked at forgiveness, shame proneness, and self-esteem in 690 LGBTQIA+ people, and found that those who had the least amount of shame and the highest amount of forgiveness had the highest levels of self-esteem.[14]

The first time I had the privilege to participate in a Gay Pride rally, I was blown away. So many people of all different orientations and gender identities were holding signs, talking, laughing, and mulling together. They were celebrating! They all seemed so comfortable and proud in their own skin. They were there to celebrate who they were. It was so beautiful and so revolutionary and so normal all at the same time that I was overcome with feelings. Why had I been so unkind to myself all this time?

—Grace, identifies as bisexual, age twenty-two

Specifically, self-forgiveness directly predicted self-esteem. Greene believes that individuals who can forgive themselves and their feelings toward others have fewer feelings of shame. This effect works to improve feelings of competency and self-worth, and increases overall self-esteem.

Greene stated, "Because shame proneness contributes to low self-esteem in LGBTQ people, we recommend helping clients to develop coping strategies to mitigate the negative impact of shame."[15]

USING AFFIRMATIONS

Once you are aware of the negative attitudes and behaviors you are still holding on to, affirmations can provide a powerful tool to start healing your self-esteem. Affirmations are short and powerful positive statements that you can repeat to yourself to challenge and replace negative thought patterns.

You can use affirmations in a variety of ways. Take some time to brainstorm a list of ten to twenty that feel meaningful to you. Think of statements that empower you and make you feel good about your strengths. Once you have a solid list of affirmations, pick five that resonate the most with you. Repeat them to yourself or say them out loud several times throughout the day. You can add calendar reminders on your phone or post a list by your mirror. The point is to repeat the positive statements often enough that you begin to form new neural pathways and rewire the way your brain works. That happens, but only if at least a small part of you knows the affirmation to be true. You can't affirm something you know to be untrue. Affirmations need to be honest and self-respecting. You can use the following list as a starting point.

- I deserve to be supported and loved.

- I'm enough, just as I am today.

- I accept my body as it is right now.

- I'm a compassionate, caring, and strong person, and I want to share those qualities with other people.

- I forgive myself for the mistakes I've made in the past.

- I have the courage to be open and vulnerable.

- Asking for help makes me stronger.

- No one, including my inner critic, has the right to make me feel unworthy.

- It's enough to just be present at the moment.

- Success is mine to define.[16]

If you find that these affirmations are too ambitious at first, it might be better to start with something like, "I will be kind to myself today." As you practice your affirmations, you'll find the ones that work best for you. Feel free to modify your list as you change and grow.

GRANT'S STORY

Grant had a difficult and unstable childhood, and only in part because he was gay. His parents separated when he was twelve after years of fighting. His father was an abusive and violent alcoholic who terrorized his mother, as well as him and his siblings. He remembers that when he realized his father had left for good, he felt that a heavy blanket had been lifted off him.

The next years weren't easy, however, as his mother attempted to care for the four kids without any financial support. She almost always worked two jobs and sometimes held three. She made sacrifices for all her kids, but she was always tired and often vacant when it came time to nurture or parent them. The area that Grant grew up in was also very traditional, closed off, and certainly homophobic. He realized early on that coming out at school or in his community would lead to bullying or even violence against him. He chose to stay in the closet for much longer than he wanted because he worried about his safety.

The first person he told, when he was seventeen, was his older sister. By then, she was living on her own and had seen more of the world, so she seemed like she might be more open. They had been very close growing up. But she did not accept him as gay. She told him that maybe it was just a phase because he was looking for a daddy that he never had. She said to him that God would not accept him as gay, so she could not. They got into a loud argument, and she threw him out of her apartment. That was a real low point for Grant. He wanted to move away from the stifling values of his town and family, but at that time, he had no means or way to move, and he hadn't even graduated high school yet. He admits that he considered suicide at that point. He had two close friends at school who, although they never talked about his being gay, he felt accepted him in some profound way that they weren't ready to talk about. Their friendship helped keep him going during those particularly dark months.

About ten months after his blowup with his sister, she texted him out of the blue and asked him to go to a movie. They both loved the cinema and had shared the same taste in movies throughout their lives. He said yes, and that was the beginning of their healing. They didn't talk about his being gay right way, but as time passed, she came to accept it. Today, she's his biggest supporter and defends him to anyone who tries to be unkind.

Grant moved away from his hometown after graduating from high school, to a much larger city in the same state. There, he says, he was able to find a gay community where he felt welcome and accepted. He is still working on his relationship with his mom, who struggles with his homosexuality, but he's grateful to have all his siblings' love and support, especially his older sister. He also still sees his two good friends from high school, who are not gay and stayed in their hometown, married, and had kids. Despite their upbringing and the pressures they might feel in their community, they are loyal and supportive of Grant as a gay man, and he enjoys being "uncle" to their kids. Grant believes that people can be educated and change because he's seen it in his own life. He believes that the power of love can change even the most stubborn minds.

As you likely know from personal experience, living in the closet is difficult, tiresome, demoralizing, and even harmful to your health. Even so, there may be some cases, especially for teens who are still dependent on their families financially and emotionally, where the disadvantages of coming out outweigh the advantages. Coming out may be especially tricky and even dangerous for LGBTQIA+ people who are a part of multiple marginalized communities.

So how do you know when it's time to come out?

WHEN TO COME OUT

It should be clear to you by now that hiding your true identity is painful and drains you of your mental and emotional resources. If you feel that the environment you live in is too hostile, however, you may decide not to come out just yet. Perhaps you need to be selective about who you come out to. That way, you have some outlet for feeling normal but can still protect yourself from the backlash you fear will follow coming out. The fact is, even most LGBTQIA+ adults are not out to everyone in every setting.[6] Although coming out has many benefits, being selective about to whom and when you come out is beneficial as well. You know that coming out opens the door to potential discrimination and victimization.

Some people live in places where being LGBTQIA+ is more accepted. It's easier for them to come out because they're more likely to get support from family and friends. Others realize their family or social environments aren't supportive and choose to wait until they're living on their own. Neither of these decisions is wrong. You decide what's best for you.

National Coming Out Day (NCOD) is an annual LGBT awareness day observed on October 11.

Regardless of the environment or society you live in, there are some points to consider to help you determine if you're ready to tell someone:

- You have come to terms with your sexuality, enough so that you can tell someone else how you view your orientation.

- You are ready to start dating and want close friends and family members to know.

- You're on the road to accepting yourself, and you're comfortable with your identity.

- You feel it is generally safe to come out.

- You're tired of hearing other people use stereotypes or negative labels in your presence.

- You feel the need to tell people about it to get it off your chest and start living freely. You might feel like you're about to explode otherwise.

BE COMFORTABLE WITH YOURSELF FIRST

Make sure you are comfortable with being queer yourself before you come out to others. If you are still questioning and not sure, it's okay to talk to a trusted friend or relative. If you're not certain that you're lesbian or bisexual, it may be hard to convince a less-than-supportive friend or relative.

Remember that you don't have to come out to everyone in your life at once. Most people come out gradually. They start by telling a counselor or a few close friends or family. A lot of people tell a counselor or therapist because they want to be sure their information stays private. Some call a LGBTQIA+ support group so they can have help working through their feelings about identity or coming out.

PART II

DEALING WITH THE CONSEQUENCES OF COMING OUT

DEALING WITH REACTIONS

*This world would be a whole lot better if we just
made an effort to be less horrible to one another.*
—Ellen Page, actress and LGBTQIA+ spokesperson

SEEKING A BETTER UNDERSTANDING

Maybe your coming out didn't go according to your hopes and plans.
It's important to remember that if people don't react the way you hope
they will, that doesn't mean you're wrong or bad, and it's not your
fault, either. You deserve to be accepted with compassion, love, and
open arms.

The previous chapter mentioned that you should be prepared for
a variety of reactions, including shock, denial, anger, guilt, sadness,
and even rejection. Whatever the case, don't write anyone off right
away. It's a good idea to give your family and friends time to accept
your truth. Although you may have been grappling with your sexual
orientation for a long time, this might be the first time they have faced
it or considered it.

This chapter discusses many of the ramifications you might have to
deal with when you come out, including how to handle it if someone
"outs" you before you're ready, how to deal with family and friends who
aren't supportive, how to keep the dialogue open with family members
who are struggling with acceptance, and how to deal with bullies and
homophobia in general.

KEEP SAFE AND HAVE A BACKUP PLAN

As mentioned in the previous chapter, have a backup plan for housing, food, school, and transportation, just in case. Find a supportive friend or relative who might allow you to crash at their house for a few days, if necessary. It helps when you have someone who can come to your rescue and offer refuge if things go wrong. If you don't have anyone close to you that fits this description, reach out to local and national LGBTQIA+ support groups like the ones discussed in this book and listed in the "Resources" section. If you find yourself homeless and with nowhere to go, you can call the LGBT National Youth Talkline at 800-246-7743 for help.

THE REACTION

When it comes to telling your parents or guardians, it may be hard for you to predict how they will react. No two families react the same way when a son or a daughter comes out of the closet.

- Your parents may have wondered about your orientation for a while and already accept it. They may even have a sense of relief that the subject is out in the open.

- Maybe your parents have reacted very negatively. They may be upset that many of their expectations for you—for example, the traditional heterosexual marriage followed by grandchildren—have suddenly disappeared. They may also negatively react because they feel that your homosexuality reflects poorly on them (and the way they raised you). Maybe they worry that you're going to hell, based on their religious beliefs. None of this is your fault.

- In some families, the reaction is split, with one parent accepting the son or daughter's announcement and the other going so far as to cut off all contact.

If you had the courage to come out to your parents or others, congratulations. The hardest part is already over—it gets better, and it gets easier throughout time. Even if your parents can never fully accept you for who you are, as time passes, they will at least get over the shock they may have initially felt and be able to move closer to establishing a functioning relationship.

Being a parent isn't easy, and the expectations your parents might have had for you are turned topsy-turvy after you come out. They may worry about your happiness and safety. It's normal for them to have some mixed emotions in the beginning. They likely carry some beliefs of heteronormativity that they learned growing up, and they may not have had much opportunity or reason to challenge those beliefs until now.

HETERONORMATIVITY

Heteronormativity is the belief that heterosexuality is the only normal and natural expression of sexuality.[1]

Keep in mind that your parents are just one possible source in which you can feel validated. You are worthy of feeling validated as a human being, no matter what kind of human being you may be. Even if you cannot count on your parents, you can still learn to love yourself.

Working with your parents and perhaps a counselor to rebuild your relationship can take a while. For all but the most extreme situations, it will be worth it to keep the door (and your heart) open to your family with the hope that they will come around.

Regardless of the reactions you get from others, try your best not to internalize them. Some people will try to change your mind, others will try to guilt-trip you, and some may treat you differently. Remember that their reactions are not a reflection of your character, but theirs. We cannot control the emotions of others; we are only in control of our own.

Don't you ever let a soul in the world
tell you that you can't be exactly who you are.
—Lady Gaga

If you are the victim of mean or hurtful comments, consider the following approaches:

- Remain calm and patient, even in the face of hurtful insults and name-calling.

- Remind yourself that you are not alone and that the problem is with the homophobic family member, not you. It is not your fault that your relative doesn't understand you. Throughout the United States—and throughout the world—there are millions of LGBTQIA+ individuals.[2]

- Keep hope that the homophobic attitude will change after your relative has had time to get used to the out-of-the-closet you. Some family members aren't homophobic deep down, they just don't know what to say or how to say it, and awkward or hurtful comments may come out of their ignorance.

- Stand up for yourself and be honest. If someone says something offensive, correct them politely with a joke. You can help these individuals learn that stereotypes aren't always accurate.

- Spend time with loving, open-minded family members during holidays or celebrations. You can build a smaller loving family unit from those who support you.

- Always remember that you can be proud of your identity.

KEEP THE DIALOGUE OPEN

You will probably find that some relationships take time to settle back to what they were. Some might change permanently. Friends and family members—even the most supportive parents—may need time to get used to your news. Stay open and patient. They may come back to you with questions time and again. Try your best to answer their questions and address their fears. It's not your job to educate them, but it might help you both anyway if you try.

If they are struggling with understanding but seem open to learning more, point them in the direction of resources especially for families of LGBTQIA+ people, for instance, PFLAG (Parents and Friends of Lesbians and Gays), at www.pflag.org.

> *I decided to tell my parents that I was gay in an e-mail. It felt like a safer way to come out to them and give them time to think about what I was saying before I saw them. I made sure I wasn't around when they would have read the e-mail. Even then, it was a long process for them to understand and accept my being gay. I let them come to me with questions and concerns when they were ready. Things are pretty good now with my parents and me.*
> —Stephanie, identifies as lesbian, age nineteen

WHEN REJECTION BECOMES ABUSIVE

Unfortunately, some LGBTQIA+ people find that homophobia is so strong and ingrained in their families that they will never change. Some family members physically or emotionally abuse their gay relatives. Many parents kick their LGBTQIA+ child out of the home when they come out. If you find yourself in an abusive situation or are out on the street, take these additional steps.

- Report any type of physical abuse to local law enforcement. There are hate crime laws in place to protect teens like you.

- Ask extended relatives, a friend's family, or a trusted teacher if you can stay with them.

- Seek shelter at one of the many LGBTQIA+ organizations that helps homeless teens find places to stay (e.g., thetrevorproject.org or nationalhomeless.org/issues/lgbt/).

- Attend counseling to deal with the pain associated with not receiving unconditional love from your family.

Living with or being related to homophobic family members can be a difficult situation. Your home is supposed to protect you from the hostile, outside world, and it is painful when you realize that family members don't accept you or are even a threat to your safety. Whether they reject you or learn to accept the real you, remember that the most important thing is that you live your life freely and stay true to yourself.

DEALING WITH HOMOPHOBIA

What is homophobia? It can be described as a fear of homosexuals, combined with loathing or disliking, based on a prejudicial negative impression one has. This book talks a lot about where these negative messages come from in our society, and you may have witnessed them in your own life.

To deal with homophobia, you should challenge your thoughts and learned beliefs first. To weed out your homophobic thoughts, you'll need to be able to recognize them as they occur. Once you have faced the negative messages that you have internalized, you're better equipped to deal with homophobic comments from others. As stated earlier, internalized homophobia harms your mental health, increasing your likelihood of suffering from depression and anxiety.[3] Various studies have backed these findings, but it also makes perfect sense. How can you be a fulfilled, happy person if you think, at some fundamental level, that you are not okay?

To challenge your thinking, take note of any uncomfortable feelings you have when confronted with gay, lesbian, or bisexual people, images, or situations. You might have thought that you were "over" these negative thoughts, but they can be buried deep. Recognizing them, calling them what they are (learned, negative, prejudiced ideas), and setting them aside can help you heal.

You need to do the work to feel comfortable in your skin. You've been bombarded with negative images and notions about gay people—conscious and subconscious—and it will take time to let those go. Letting go is good, healthy work that's worth doing. If you can afford a counselor, seeing someone who understands or specializes in LGBTQIA+ issues can help ease the process. Check your area for LGBTQIA+-focused counseling.

The next question is, Are you responsible for countering every homophobic remark you hear as you make your way in the world? Is it your job to educate the uneducated in your life and circle? The answer is no. It might give you a feeling of pride and accomplishment to do so in certain circumstances. Sticking up for yourself is a very self-loving thing to do. Rather than take on the entire world, it's probably healthier to focus on the people who matter in your life—family and friends.

So, how can you combat homophobic remarks from family and friends? Consider these points.

- Remind yourself that homophobia is usually based on a lack of knowledge on the topic and that they are only repeating stereotypes and opinions they have been exposed to in their environment. This is especially true if someone is raised in a conservative or religious family.

- Educate yourself on why someone is homophobic. For example, some people have never knowingly had a friendship with a gay person and simply do not understand homosexuality, while others may be secretly ashamed of their homosexual desires.

- Be realistic and realize that someone's homophobia will not disappear overnight or in one conversation.

- Use logic, statistics, and facts when defending gay rights.

Sometimes the decision of whether to stand up for yourself or let an insult pass is an easy one. More often, it's complicated and painful. If you stand by silently, you may find later that the situation gnaws at you. Silence comes at a cost; however, trying to counter and educate every time you're confronted with a homophobic remark would be exhausting and maybe even dangerous.

Homophobia isn't likely to go away in our society any time soon, and confronting it is no small feat. You'll probably be dealing with some form of it your entire life. It's a war with many battles. Remember that a sign of a healthy mental state is when you can let go of the things you cannot change. Focus on what you can control, which is how you feel about and treat yourself. That may include needing to stick up for yourself at times.

The best advice I've read about this issue comes from Anne Dohrenwend, Ph.D., in her book *Coming Around*:

> Please remember that you did not cause these problems. Any perceived inadequacies related to your ability to explain or defend yourself are not a function of being less than the one who attacks you, but, instead, a function of being asked to perform remarkably, over and over, in stressful situations. Be gentle with yourself. Don't expect to say the right thing at the right time every time you are presented with bias. This would be asking too much from yourself and would distract you from your job, which is to be happy. In the end, there is no better response to homophobia than to resist being derailed by it. Live your life shamelessly and passionately.[4]

HOMOPHOBIC BULLYING

Bullying, which is the act of trying to harm, threaten, intimidate, or humiliate someone who you have perceived power over, continues to be a serious problem in this country for many school-age youths. While any student can be at risk for bullying for a variety of reasons, LGBTQIA+ students are at a much higher risk for being the target of verbal slurs and physical attacks, whether at school or online. The Human Rights Campaign's "2018 LGBTQ Youth Report" found the following alarming trends when they surveyed LGBTQIA+ teens:

- Only 26 percent said they always feel safe in their school classrooms.

from being bullied by students, teachers, and school staff based on sexual orientation and gender identity.[6]

Become familiar with nondiscrimination laws. These laws also can help. At this time, only thirteen states and the District of Columbia have school nondiscrimination laws and statewide regulations to protect LGBTQIA+ students from discrimination in schools based on sexual orientation and gender identity, including being unfairly denied access to facilities, sports teams, and clubs.[7]

Find out how you can start a GSA club if your school doesn't have one. The Centers for Disease Control and Prevention (CDC) encourages schools to create gay-affirming groups like GSAs and use health education criteria that are LGBTQIA+ inclusive.[8]

Ultimately, it is the school administration's job to provide a safe ace for all students to learn. But you may be able to help that process

CYBERSTALKING AND CYBERBULLYING

LGBTQIA+ youth report much higher rates of digital dating abuse and cyberbullying than heterosexual youth. Less than 10 percent of them seek help and rarely from parents or teachers.[9] Cyberstalking and cyberbullying include such acts as sending unwanted, frightening, or offensive e-mails, text messages, or instant messages; harassing and threatening on social media; tracking computer and internet use; and using GPS to track a person.

If you're a victim of cyberstalking or cyberbullying, first, don't respond to any of the messages. Block the person who is cyberbullying you and keep all of the evidence. Record dates, times, and descriptions of the incidents. Save and print screenshots, e-mails, text messages, and so on. You can use this evidence to report cyberbullying to web providers and cell phone service providers, as well as the police. Stalking and threats of violence are crimes. You are protected under the law from such violence and intimidation.

- Just 5 percent said all of their teachers and school staff are
  ive of LGBTQIA+ people.

- Only 13 percent reported hearing positive messages ab
  LGBTQIA+ in school.

This report showed that bullying is still rampant in many sch
you're an LGBTQIA+ student:

- Seventy-three percent of LGBTQIA+ youth repor
  the target of verbal threats because of their actual or
  LGBTQIA+ identity.

- Thirty percent received physical threats because of their L(
  identity.

- Forty-three percent had been bullied on school prope
  twelve months of taking the survey.[5]

What can be done? Several measures have been proven t

- *Locate a formal system of support, for example LGBTQ*
  Teens who have access to such LGBTQIA+ clubs as a Ga
  Alliance (GSA) find that belonging to these formal
  support can mitigate negative experiences, reduce risky
  and reduce stress. These clubs use positive peer pressure
  age harassment.

- *Find a teacher who you feel would be supportive or already*
  to be an ally when it comes to sexual orientation issues an
  to support your GSA. They can become a source of help
  as well.

- *Get to know the antibullying laws.* These laws have been
  work; however, only nineteen states, the District of Colt
  Puerto Rico have antibullying laws to protect LGBTQIA

along by forming a cohesive group and raising these issues together. Studies show that positive exposure to LGBTQIA+ individuals dramatically reduces homophobia.[10]

In high school, I was teased and called "fag" and "homo" repeatedly, sometimes right in front of teachers, who did nothing. My only solace was art class, where I found more open-minded people. None of my regular bullies were in the art classes, either. I felt more free there.
—Steve, identifies as gay, age twenty

DEALING WITH BULLIES

Bullying is harmful to everyone. It makes a school a place of fear and can lead to more stress and violence for everyone. The following are some tactics for dealing with a bully:

- *Be confident.* Standing tall to someone who wants to intimidate you takes the wind out of their sails. They often lose their power when you don't cower to their bullying.

- *Stay connected.* Bullies try to make their victims feel alone and powerless. When you have a support group, you'll be armed with confidence and can reclaim your power after a negative interaction with a bully.

- *Use unemotional language.* Be assertive, but don't challenge a bully.

- *Keep a record of the comments or behavior.* If you are being bullied online or via social media, take screenshots and keep them as evidence to show your parents, the school, or the police.

- *Get an ally.* If you know this bully is always in a particular area of the school, have friends come with you when you may run into this person. You can also return the favor if needed.

ERIC'S STORY

When Eric came out to his parents, he was thirteen. Pretty young. When pressed to tell them which girl at school he liked, he told them that he liked boys, not girls. They immediately put him in therapy. His mother wondered what she had done wrong. They told him he would grow out of the feelings. They also said things like, "You play sports and are athletic; you can't be gay," "Sometimes we just find people's personalities fun and attractive, but you shouldn't confuse that with romantic feelings," and "You're just under stress and don't understand your feelings."

Their reactions were hurtful to Eric. He was young and believed that his parents knew better about most things than he did. It caused him to question his feelings and thoughts. At the heart of that, he heard the message, "You are not okay if you are this way."

Ironically, what ended up helping Eric was a counselor his parents had him see. Not the first one he saw, but a later one. By that time, he was fifteen. He immediately felt "okay" with this counselor and found it easy to trust her. Slowly, she helped him come to terms with being gay and who he was. Her mantra to him was, "You have to accept yourself before anyone else can accept you."

Now eighteen, Eric lives "mostly" out, he says. His parents have tacitly accepted his lifestyle. They see he is happier than he ever had been before (they've told him this). They haven't fully embraced him as gay, but Eric has faith that they will. He does believe that you have to accept yourself first before you can bring anyone who's struggling along with you. He has lived it. His advice to others is to remember that your loved ones' first reactions to your coming out are likely not where they'll end up. If they reject you or your lifestyle, give them time. They might be surprised and hurt by the news at first. Give them time to come around.

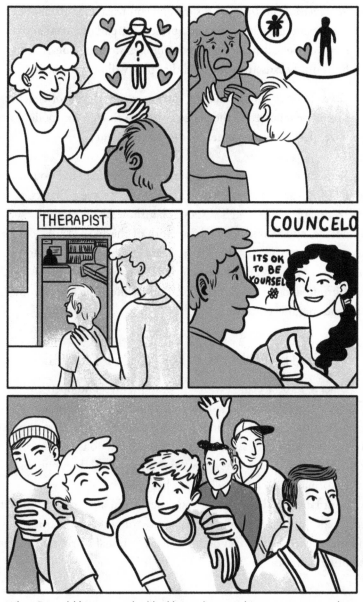

When Eric told his parents he liked boys, they sent him to see a counselor. His counselor taught him it was okay to accept himself. *Illustration by Kate Haberer*

- *Tell someone you trust.* Find someone you trust and talk about what is happening to you. Teachers, principals, parents, or sympathetic relatives can all help. Sometimes bullies stop as soon as an adult finds out because they're afraid that they will be punished.

- *Take it seriously.* If the bullying spills over into threats or violence, it should be reported to the police as a hate crime. Many police forces have specialist units to deal with these incidents.

Remember that you don't deserve to be bullied, and you are not alone. Most people don't hate LGBTQIA+ people. Thanks to the media, organizations, and TV shows that show likable and upstanding gay people, and thanks to the hard work of the LGBTQIA+ community, which has worked so hard to be heard and understood, many more youth today have been exposed to positive gay role models. Attitudes are shifting, and homophobia is on the decline. You have more allies than you might even realize.

THE JOURNEY TO ACCEPTANCE

You deserve to be accepted with compassion, love, and open arms. Part of the process of accepting and loving yourself is working hard to not internalize the hurtful comments and reactions you get from others. That's not always easy. Remember that these reactions are not a reflection of your character. They are a reflection of the homophobic and heteronormative society in which we live.

Your family will always love you. They might also come around and accept you just the way you are. The only thing you have control over and the only thing you can do is the hard, internal work of loving and accepting yourself.

CHAPTER FIVE

BUILDING A SUPPORT NETWORK

I've been embraced by a new community. That's what happens when you're finally honest about who you are; you find others like you.
—Chaz Bono, writer, musician, and actor

SEEKING A BETTER UNDERSTANDING

As this book mentions, coming out is usually a multistep process that happens in phases. It's totally up to you who you decide to tell and when. Start with people you think will support and accept you. They can be the kernel of creating a supportive network.

Remember to give your family and friends time to accept your truth. They may not be on board immediately or be able to support you right away actively, but they may be willing to help you find support from other sources. Maybe your mom or dad isn't yet ready to fly a rainbow flag, for example, but they may be willing to drive you to the local LGBTQIA+ meeting so you can start finding people who understand and support you.

This chapter discusses some of the ways you can start to build the support and friendship you need to survive school and be your true self. Everyone's journey is different, and everyone's personal and cultural situations are different. There are people who will understand you, no matter where you live. The methods and advice in this chapter aren't for everyone. You shouldn't feel pressured to start or join a group if it doesn't feel right at this time. Find the approach that's comfortable for you—being kind to and supportive of yourself and patient on your journey.

START SMALL

One friend, one ally, one supportive teacher, one understanding relative, one online connection. One is all you need at first. If you feel it's appropriate, start at your school. Does it have a club or support group already in place? Even if you aren't ready to join it just yet (or ever), identifying people in that group is a great way to find like-minded teens and adults.

If the climate at your school is unwelcoming to or even hostile toward LGBTQIA+ people and issues, you may feel more comfortable looking at the wider community or online at safe and supportive places. This chapter covers some of the options.

START LOCAL

The simplest way to start is to check your school to see if they have any support groups or alliances for LGBTQIA+ students. If you don't feel comfortable starting this process at school, you can start by searching for groups in your area. Search for "LGBT support groups near me" or "LGBT organizations near me." If you visit CenterLink at www.lgbtcenters.org/LGBTCenters, you can enter your address or ZIP code and instantly see groups close to where you live. GLAAD (Gay and Lesbian Alliance against Defamation) provides a helpful list of resources at www.glaad.org/resourcelist. The resources are organized by interest, and the links take you right to that particular organization's LGBTQIA+-related offers.

Spending some time online to find a group near you is a great way to build connections and friendships with people who can relate to what you're going through. In addition to LGBTQIA+ support groups, also consider pride parades, rallies, and festivals.

ONLINE SUPPORT

Whether or not you have support in your community, the internet is filled with excellent, supportive resources that can address every question and issue you could ever have. Having the resources and support you need to navigate being a LGBTQIA+ teenager can start online. In addition to CenterLink and GLAAD, check out these sources of support.

Gay, Lesbian, and Straight Education Network (GLSEN)
www.glsen.org

You'll see that GLSEN is referenced numerous times in this chapter. That's because the organization specifically works to ensure that LGBTQIA+ students can learn and grow in a school environment free from bullying and harassment. It was founded in 1990, by a group of teachers. The site contains loads of information and references to help with various school issues.

It Gets Better Project
itgetsbetter.org

The It Gets Better Project inspires people throughout the world to share their stories and remind the next generation of LGBTQIA+ youth that hope is out there and it will get better.

Q Card Project
www.qcardproject.com

The Q Card is an easy-to-use communication tool to empower LGBTQIA+ youth to become actively engaged in their health and support the people who provide their care.

Q Chat Space
www.qchatspace.org

Q Chat Space is a digital LGBTQIA+ center where teens can join live chat, professionally facilitated online support groups.

Bisexual Resource Center
biresource.org

Since 1985, the Bisexual Resource Center has been committed to providing support to the bisexual community and raising public awareness about bisexuality and bisexual people.

The Trevor Project
www.thetrevorproject.org

The Trevor Project is a national organization that provides crisis intervention and suicide prevention services to LGBTQIA+ people age twenty-five and younger.[1] Their TrevorSpace.org site calls itself an "affirming international community for LGBTQIA+ young people ages thirteen to twenty-four." Join it to make connections with people throughout the world.

Parents and Friends of Lesbians and Gays (PFLAG)
www.pflag.org

The first and largest organization for LGBTQIA+ people and their parents, families, and allies, PFLAG was founded in 1973, as the simple act of a mother publicly supporting her gay son. If your parents or loved ones are asking questions and trying to understand or find a way to support you, this organization's website is a good place to send them.

JOIN/CREATE A GSA CLUB

Research has shown that GSAs (Gay–Straight Alliances) improve school climate, individual well-being, and educational outcomes for LGBTQIA+ youth.[2] Participation in GSAs is related to feelings of positive school connectedness and improved academic achievement for LGBTQIA+ youth, and regardless of whether LGBTQIA+ students participate in their school's GSA, just having a GSA in their school can create a more positive school climate for LGBTQIA+ students.[3]

If you're interested in starting a GSA club yourself, this section can help you figure out where to start and what to do. The GSA

MORE ABOUT THE TREVOR PROJECT

The Trevor Project isn't just about crisis intervention and suicide prevention. It also provides such programs and services as a handbook for coming out, support centers throughout the country, educational materials for LGBTQIA+ youth and their loved ones, and Trevor mentors and ambassadors. It is also committed to providing important research on the lives of LGBTQIA+ youth that's hard to find elsewhere. Figure 5.1 shows the many ways you can contact them.

The Trevor Project was founded in 1998, by the creators of the Academy Award–winning short film *Trevor*. It's a sixteen-minute film that you can watch at https://www.thetrevorproject.org/about/history-film/ or on YouTube at https://www.youtube.com/watch?v=CO5uKgTETSI.

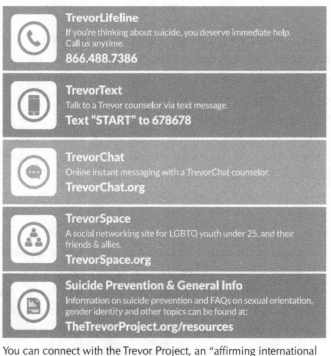

TrevorLifeline
If you're thinking about suicide, you deserve immediate help.
Call us anytime.
866.488.7386

TrevorText
Talk to a Trevor counselor via text message.
Text "START" to 678678

TrevorChat
Online instant messaging with a TrevorChat counselor.
TrevorChat.org

TrevorSpace
A social networking site for LGBTQ youth under 25, and their friends & allies.
TrevorSpace.org

Suicide Prevention & General Info
Information on suicide prevention and FAQs on sexual orientation, gender identity and other topics can be found at:
TheTrevorProject.org/resources

You can connect with the Trevor Project, an "affirming international community for LGBTQIA+ young people ages thirteen to twenty-four." Join it to make connections with people throughout the world.
The Trevor Project, West Hollywood, CA

Network, at gsanetwork.org, also has lots of resources. You can search for a GSA in your area from the site or register your own GSA with their organization. They also provide ideas and suggestions for things to do at your meetings.

GSAs AND THE LAW

If you attend a public school that has other noncurricular clubs, the Equal Access Act states that your school cannot deny the formation of a GSA. This federal law also says that schools cannot treat GSAs differently from other noncurricular clubs, so if the Chess Club gets to advertise on the morning announcements and hang up posters in the hallways, the GSA does, too.

The American Civil Liberties Union (ACLU) works to protect and ensure the civil rights of all people and has offices throughout the country. Visit www.aclu.org to find an ACLU chapter near you. The ACLU has helped many students who have been told they could not have a GSA.

After searching for a while, I became discouraged. If groups were out there, they were hard to find. My high school didn't have a LGBT support group, so after lots of worrying and thinking, I decided to try to start one on my own. In the first meeting, two people came! We sat in the classroom and exchanged stories for an hour. In the next meeting, four people came. Some were straight and wanted to be allies. We changed the name of the club to the Gay–Straight Alliance, and more people joined. During the next school year, I became the unofficial president of this club. We did a lot of education about body image issues, great role models, gender identity, overcoming isolation, and more. It really helped me feel connected and not so alone. I think it helped other students, too.

—Michael, identifies as gay, age eighteen

STEPS FOR STARTING A GSA AT YOUR SCHOOL

These steps were adapted from the Gay, Lesbian, and Straight Education Network's (GLSEN) suggestions on their website,[4] but you can find lots of different ways to reach the same goal from other like-minded organizations. Use these steps as a guide and check with your school to see if they have a preferred way to develop a club before you get too deep in the weeds. Note that most schools treat GSAs as an extracurricular student-led club, much like the Chess Club, the Science Bowl, or the Photography Club.

1. *Follow your school guidelines.* A GSA is like any other extracurricular student-led club that your school has, so you need to follow the school guidelines for setting it up. Look in your student handbook or online at your school's site for rules regarding clubs. You may have to formally appeal to your school's administration and fulfill specific administrative requirements. Sometimes you might need to write bylaws or file a petition. Learn your school's regulations ahead of time so you can be sure to follow them correctly.

2. *Find a faculty advisor.* This person could be a teacher or other faculty member. Look for someone who would be supportive of your cause and goals or who has already shown themselves to be allies.

3. *Tell the school administration.* Let administrators know right away that you want to create a GSA club. It can be beneficial to have them on your side. They can work as liaisons to teachers, parents, community members, and the school board. If an administrator opposes the GSA, provide them information from www.glsen.org/gsa.

4. *Find other students to join.* Invite fellow students who are interested in building an affirming LGBTQIA+ space. One place to

start is to check with existing clubs for students who might have an interest. Try to recruit a broad base of members. You should aim to have at least ten people per meeting, which will generally mean a group of thirty or so members with sporadic involvement or a group of ten to fifteen members who are consistently committed. Your advisor might also have ideas of students who may be interested.

5. *Find a meeting place.* It will probably be on school grounds, but check the school guidelines for information on extracurricular student-led clubs, which should mention where meetings are typically held (on campus or somewhere else). You may want to find a meeting place within the school that offers some level of privacy yet is still easily accessible. You may decide that you want to meet in a visible space to enhance the presence of your club at your school.

6. *Get the word out.* There are many ways to let students know about your organization. Use a combination of the school bulletin, announcements, flyers, and word of mouth. Get creative through visuals that register with LGBTQIA+ people, like rainbows and trans flags.

7. *Plan the first meeting.* Organize your meeting from start to finish to get the most out of your time. There are many things you can do, including having discussions, inviting speakers, holding workshops, playing games, and providing food or snacks. Many suggestions are described in the GLSEN Jump-Start Guide at https://eqfl.org/sites/default/files/Jumpstart1.pdf.

8. *Hold your first meeting.* It's a good idea to start the meeting with a discussion about why people think the group is needed or important. You can also think about projects that your club could during the year, as well as determine the topics you want to discuss at the meetings.

9. *Establish community agreements.* Creating basic ground rules will help every member feel safe. Group discussions should always be confidential and respectful.

10. *Plan for the future.* Develop an action plan and a calendar of events and projects. What are the club's goals for the next year or years? Use the resources mentioned in this section to help.

GLSEN'S DAY OF SILENCE

GLSEN's Day of Silence is a national student-led protest where participants take a vow of silence to highlight the silencing and erasure of LGBTQIA+ people in schools. This event, usually held on a Friday in April, is something your GSA could do together. Students in middle school through college participate. Those who sign up for the Day of Silence hand out cards to others explaining their silence and why they have chosen not to talk.

COMMUNITY GSA

If your school is not supportive, another good option is to start a community GSA for students/teens in your town. This group would not be associated with a single school, so you would need to find a separate meeting place, for instance, the local library or other community space. One benefit of this approach is that you have a larger pool of potential members from which to draw. With social media, it's easier now more than ever to find and connect with students at nearby high schools.

In terms of the future, your goal should be that the GSA club becomes sustainable enough that it will continue to run even after you've graduated or moved on. Part of that is finding a teacher or other faculty member to serve as your club's advisor. This person should be dedicated to the club, enough so that they can help sustain the club after you've left. If you do this right, the club will be your legacy to your school.

OTHER WAYS TO FIND SUPPORT

If the idea of joining or starting a GSA club seems ludicrous to you based on where you live, you can find companionship and support in other ways:

- *Performing arts department:* School theater and choir departments sometimes have more open-minded people who are more likely to accept you as you are. If you don't have acting or singing talent, you can help out behind the scenes.

STEVE'S STORY

When Steve told his parents he thought he was gay, his dad immediately responded, "Think again." They told him that he needed to "shape up" or he would have to move out of their house and live elsewhere. He was fifteen.

In addition to feeling alienated from the cishet society he lived in, he was now alienated from his parents. He was also mocked and bullied at school. Although he never fully came out to anyone at school, the students seemed to sense that he was different. He was teased and called "fag" and "homo" repeatedly, sometimes right in front of teachers, who did nothing. His only solace was art class, where he found more interesting and open-minded people.

Steve endured punishment and rejection for most of his high school years. It wasn't until he went away to a small liberal arts college to study art that he found a group of allies and even gay people like him. His college years have been so much better and more fulfilling. He is also in therapy to deal with the years of being harassed and shamed for who he is. To any gay teen who will listen, he says hang in there. It gets so much better. His life is now interesting, fulfilling, and filled with people who love and care for him, just the way he is.

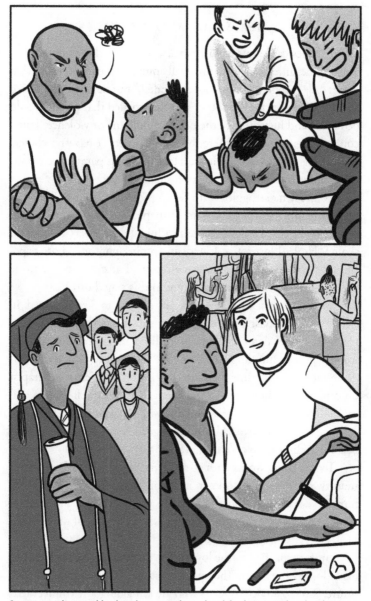

Steve was alienated both at home and at school for his sexuality, but he was able to be himself when he moved to college. *Illustration by Kate Haberer*

JAMES: OUT AND PROUD

When James came out to his parents, which he did to them both at the same time, they were unusually quiet. His parents were what James calls "progressive and open-minded," but he was still worried about telling them. His mother said she worried that his life would be harder and he would be the target of bullying or violence. James couldn't argue with her there, but he told her, "I have no choice, Mom. This is who I am." He feels lucky that his parents were basically supportive and accepting of his being queer.

Even so, he struggled with feelings of self-doubt and lack of self-worth during his teen years. Perhaps that was normal for all teenagers, he told himself. Underneath it all, there was a feeling of shame. He had lost a few friends in coming out, and those experiences weighed on him. He was already an anxious and neurotic kid, as he tells it, and being different in this way didn't help.

When he got to college, James started to get involved in LGBTQIA+ activist groups. At first, this was something he did to "meet guys." After a while, he realized they were doing really important and fulfilling work, and he was glad to be a part of it. At about that same time, he started seeing an inexpensive therapist on campus. By then he was ready to face his poor self-esteem and make different choices. His therapist was fantastic and helped him "change his perspective." He also changed his major and decided to become a clinical psychologist himself.

Today, James works with at-risk teens in the LGBTQIA+ community. He loves his work. In addition to helping teens just like him make it through those rough years, their stories of bravery and courage have also made him even prouder to be part of the resilient LGBTQIA+ community.

James is married to the love of his life, and he and his husband just adopted their son. They plan on adding to their family in the future. James's advice to teens who are struggling: "If you feel that you are alone, please know in your heart that the LGBTQIA+ community is everywhere, and we are here to support you."

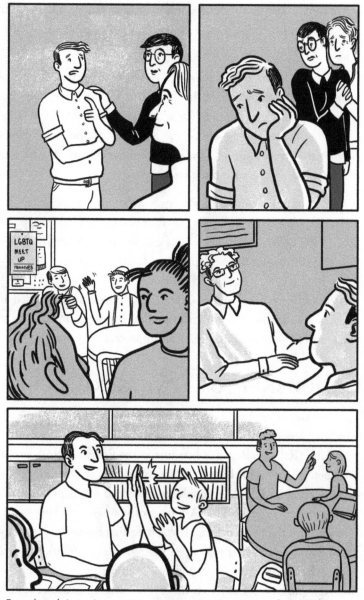

Even though James's parents were supportive, James struggled with his self-worth throughout school. He started to see a therapist and joined LGBTQIA+ activist groups, helping him find his confidence and passion for helping LGBTQIA+ youth. *Illustration by Kate Haberer*

- *Art classes:* The same goes for many artistic people. You may find support and friendship in the art and pottery classes and events at your school.

- *Progressive churches and religions:* If you're Christian, check out the local Episcopal, Unitarian, Quaker, or Lutheran church. If you're Jewish, many individual synagogues welcome LGBTQIA+ members. You should check the websites of the local church/synagogue before you go (for words like "welcoming"). Check out www.gaychurch.org for more resources.

- *Local progressive political party organizations:* Check out the local youth political groups that are friendly toward and supportive of LGBTQIA+ individuals, for example, the National Stonewall Young Democrats or the Republican Unity Coalition.

Look for other friends, teens, or adults who are open-minded and accepting. Starting with one person or one connection can help you branch out to an entire community of supporters.

THE JOURNEY TO A LOVING COMMUNITY

What does the future hold in our country for LGBTQIA+ people? The general trend seems to be moving in a positive direction. A recent study by the Public Religion Research Institute found that younger Americans are 17 percent more likely than older Americans to say they support laws protecting LGBTQIA+ people from various forms of discrimination.[5] Moreover, more LGBTQIA+ Americans are involved in or part of support groups than ever before.[6] If you're feeling isolated in your small town or community where many people aren't accepting, it's important to realize that the country, in general, is becoming more accepting. Your reality right now may feel much more discouraging than the statistics and trends tell us.

I moved away from my hometown after graduating from high school because of a job. It was a much larger city in the same state. To start with, I joined a welcoming church and met friends there. Throughout time, I was able to build a sizeable gay community where I felt welcomed and accepted.
—Grant, identifies as gay, age twenty-two

Humans crave connection with others, and you are no exception. We all need meaningful connections with others who love and accept us. If you have just started coming out to others in your life and met resistance, it might feel like you will never have the luxury of such meaningful connections. If you believe nothing else, you must agree that statistically, you will find a safe place where you can be yourself with others who accept you. Many, many other LGBTQIA+ teens have come through the fog to the other side, to find their loving, accepting communities. It might take some work and some time, but it's worth it. It does get better.

PART III

RESOLUTION

CHAPTER SIX

SEX AND LOVE

The power of love is that it sees all people.
—DaShanne Stokes, author, sociologist, public speaker, and pundit

SEEKING A BETTER UNDERSTANDING

It's a big step when you're at the point where you want to think about romantic relationships and sex. You probably feel comfortable enough with yourself and your orientation at this point that you're ready to share a special bond with another person. To put yourself out there and risk being hurt is courageous, but being loved is also a crucial need of the human condition. You deserve happiness and love, so good for you.

This chapter discusses the issues of sex and love from the queer perspective, including such topics as first dates, breakups, bringing home partners to meet your family, safe sex, STIs, and consent. It could never attempt to cover every question you have or address every issue out there, so we've included trusted links in the "Resources" section, where you can get more information. Following this book's approach, this chapter does not cover transgender sex, other than in a broad sense. Many of the sections can be helpful to any teen, regardless of orientation or gender.

LOVE, RELATIONSHIPS, AND RESPECT

Before you ever consider having sex with someone you've been seeing, it's important to make sure the relationship is healthy and respectful on both ends. Maybe you're not in a relationship yet but you're wondering how it would look. This section covers some things to ask for, some things you should expect to give back in a relationship, and warning signs.

Consider these signs of a healthy relationship, which apply whether it's a friendship or a romantic relationship. Your partner should do the following:

- Respect your boundaries.

- Respect your chosen gender pronouns or name.

- Give you space to hang out with other people (friends and family) without becoming jealous.

- Never threaten to "out" you to other people.

- Never insult you, be overly critical, or try to intimidate you.

A healthy relationship is a partnership where each person gives and receives. There is space, trust, and respect for differences in a healthy relationship. While in a relationship, you should have activities and interests apart from your partner, and you should maintain your other relationships with friends and family.

Your partner should accept you as you are and not try to change you. Of course, you should return respect and follow these behavioral guidelines as well.

SIGNS OF AN UNHEALTHY RELATIONSHIP

Violence in any form is a huge red flag. It's not the only important sign of an unhealthy relationship, although it's a significant one. You may be in an unhealthy relationship when one (or both) of you does any of the following:

- Is overly controlling, makes all the decisions, and tries to tell the other what they can or cannot do.

- Is entirely dependent on the other or loses their identity.

- Is aggressive, starts fights, or is dishonest.

- Is disrespectful, makes fun of the other, or crosses boundaries.

- Intimidates or tries to control the other using fear.

- Engages in physical or sexual violence.[1]

> *You know, it's funny; when you look at someone through*
> *rose-colored glasses, all the red flags just look like flags.*
> —Wanda the Owl, from *BoJack Horseman*, Season 2

Not all of these issues are equally catastrophic. You may be able to talk to your partner about a disrespectful attitude they sometimes have, for example. If one of you becomes too dependent on the other, you can try to discuss it. If you are both able to talk honestly about your feelings *and* you can ask for what you need, you can work together to improve things. See the section later in this chapter about how to ask for what you need in a relationship.

Violence, intimidation, outright hostility, and dishonesty should be deal-breakers. You deserve better than that. If you are the one exhibiting these behaviors, it's time to dig deep and deal with your issues, preferably with a certified counselor.

DATING VIOLENCE

Hopefully, you'll never find yourself in a violent dating relationship, but many teens do. One of the only studies on LGBTQIA+ teens, released by the Urban Institute, showed significantly higher rates of dating violence among LGBTQIA+ youth. While 29 percent of heterosexual youth surveyed reported being physically abused by dating partners, for example, 42.8 percent of LGBTQIA+ youth reported abuse. The rate of sexual victimization for LGBTQIA+ respondents was 23 percent, which is almost double heterosexual youth, of whom 12.3 percent reported sexual coercion. Transgender youth reported the highest rates, with 88.9 percent reporting physical dating violence. This study also showed that LGBTQIA+ youth were much more likely than their heterosexual peers to be perpetrators of dating violence.[2]

This information is not here to depress you or make you weary of all possible dates and partners, but to make you aware that it does happen. If it happens to you, you can better recognize the signs. Dating violence can be emotional, physical, or sexual.

- *Emotional violence* involves name-calling, behaving in a controlling or jealous way, always keeping tabs on the other person, shaming, and bullying.

- *Physical violence* involves such injury or trauma as pinching, hitting, shoving, punching, kicking, and so on. Physical violence also includes forcing someone to consume alcohol or use drugs.

- *Sexual violence* involves forcing a partner to have sex or engage in sexual activities when they do not or cannot consent, either physical or nonphysical. An example of nonphysical sexual violence is if someone were to threaten to out you unless you engaged in sex with them.

If you have been a victim of dating violence in any form, you should end the relationship. Keep any evidence you have of the violence or threats, for example, e-mails, texts, photos, letters, and so on. Take pictures of bruises and other bodily harm. Go to a trusted adult or friend for help, especially if you feel that you are still in danger or may be stalked or threatened. Unfortunately, you may find that you have fewer survivor resources and little support from your family and friends, which makes it hard to find good help. In that case, there are online resources like www.breakthecycle.org and www.loveisrespect.org that can help you. You can call 1-866-331-9474, chat online, or text "loveis" to 22522 to speak to someone. For help with cyberstalking or online bullying, see the box entitled "Cyberstalking and Cyberbullying" in chapter 4.

ASKING FOR WHAT YOU NEED

Asking for what you need in a relationship can be difficult, especially if you've grown up in an environment that consistently diminished your needs, wishes, or opinions. It's hard to do because you have to be vulnerable, and you risk hurting your partner's feelings.

Asking for what you want in your relationship will help grow your sense of empowerment and self-worth. If you aren't consistently able to ask for or get what you need, resentment, disconnection, and misunderstanding can grow.

You are worthy of having your needs met. Do some self-reflection about what your needs are. You may have an overall feeling of discontent but aren't sure why. You need to do the work to figure out and articulate, as best you can, what you need that you feel you aren't getting.

Pick a time to sit down with your partner when you are both relaxed—not upset or stressed—and explain everything. Express what you need more of and *why* it's something you need in the relationship. Don't blame or accuse them; instead, focus on "I" sentences (e.g., "I feel more connected to you when your phone is put away when we're having good talks"). In turn, be open to your partner voicing their needs. Relationships are a two-way street, and both parties deserve to feel supported, loved, and respected.

HOW TO DEAL WITH FIRST DATES

First dates can be both exciting and fraught with nerves and tension. You're probably putting a lot of hopes on this one date with this person, and that can result in the date not going so well. The first step is to lower your expectations. Think of it as a way to spend a few hours getting to know someone who might or might not end up being a friend. Whatever happens, you have met a friend, found a romance, or learned what you don't like in other people.

Prepare for the worst but expect the best. That means picking a location that allows you to spend one-on-one time (no movies), yet will enable you to conclude the date in a comfortable fashion (get coffee or ice cream together, not a full dinner where you might have to wait awkwardly for the bill). Be real, that is, be yourself. Trust and follow your feelings.

If you're like the rest of humanity, you'll probably have to go on a lot of first dates before you click with someone. Treat these experiences as training and learn how to be yourself, and be open and caring to others.

INTRODUCING YOUR PARTNER TO YOUR FAMILY

It's a big step when you feel like you're ready to introduce your special someone to important people in your life. If you are ready, the first two questions to ask yourself are is your family truly ready and is your partner "game"?

Make sure your partner is clued in about your family dynamics, and be honest. Tell them what kind of response they can expect from your family and where your family is in their journey to accepting you. Also, are there certain subjects that they should avoid? Be as specific as possible. Don't keep secrets from them, even if it means admitting, for example, that your dad is outwardly homophobic and might say something insensitive or insulting. The more prepared your partner is, the better it will go.

You should also prepare your family. If your family is still coming to terms with your out status, you may need to give them more time. If this is the first romantic partner your family will meet, give them a heads-up to ensure that everyone is on the same page. Make sure they realize how important that first meeting is to you. Answer any questions they may have and be patient about listening to their concerns.

Thanksgiving or holiday get-togethers are not the best times to bring your partner into the family fray. Instead, pick a casual setting.

Some good examples include an outdoor cafe, a local coffee house, or a neighborhood restaurant where you feel comfortable. First meetings are better when they aren't long. When in doubt, keep it simple, casual, and short.

It might be smart to agree on a safe word (or phrase), too, which, when spoken, means "meet me in the bathroom" or "let's get out of here" (or whatever you choose). That can be a way for your partner to pull the plug if they are feeling super uncomfortable.

Finally, don't be afraid to show your family how happy you are, in as natural a way as possible. But don't force anything. Seeing you happy could help your family learn to accept and support you.

DEALING WITH BREAKUPS

You can't get over a breakup unless you allow yourself to feel all the feelings, as horrible as they seem at the time. Don't turn to using drugs or alcohol, engaging in one-night stands, medicating, or other ways of avoiding or ignoring the pain. You'll just end up with another, much bigger problem and still be left with the pain of the breakup as well. Give yourself time to mourn and cry. Crying is therapeutic.

Disconnect yourself from your ex. Block your ex's social media accounts and avoid places where they are if you can. Separating yourself is a healthy and important step in moving on.

Then go out and be your own person. Go out and do what you feel like doing. See friends, go for a run or to the gym, see a movie by yourself. Were there things you loved that your former partner didn't like to do with you? Go. Do. Those. Things. You get to think about you, and only you, for a little bit. The point is to regain your feeling of independence. It's a great time to try new things, too. Try a new sport, play an instrument, write a story, volunteer at the animal shelter.

Don't isolate yourself. Reach out to supportive family and friends. You don't have to tell them all the nitty-gritty details of your breakup if you don't feel comfortable doing so. Just being around your family and friends while they are doing their usual thing can help lift your spirits.

Unfortunately, breakups are a part of life. They are painful, but you will survive. If you learn from the relationship, your next one can be even better.

INTIMACY AND SEX

Traditional sex education, when available, focuses on puberty education for cisgender people, heterosexual sex, pregnancy prevention, and prevention of sexually transmitted infections (STIs). Traditional sex education and safe-sex guides don't reflect or provide information about same-sex and queer relationships. They are usually based on the assumption that everyone's gender (male, female, nonbinary, trans) is the same as the sex they were assigned at birth (male, female, intersex, or differences in sexual development).

If you saw any LGBTQIA+ representation in your health education class, you are part of only 5 percent of U.S. teens, according to the Gay, Lesbian, and Straight Education Network's 2015 National School Climate Survey.[3] Homophobia and transphobia have prevented most schools and organizations from even acknowledging the existence of LGBTQIA+ and nonbinary individuals.

Things are slowly shifting, however. There are also a lot of good resources online, so the answers are out there—you just might have to go digging. For a full description of gender and sexual identities as they are understood at this time, refer to the tables in chapter 1.

There's this illusion that homosexuals have sex and heterosexuals fall in love. That's completely untrue. Everybody wants to be loved.
—Boy George, singer, songwriter, and fashion designer

TYPES OF SEX

It's time for the "sex talk," one you probably didn't get from school or maybe your parents. The focus of this section is on not only the variations of sex that human beings can enjoy, but also being informed enough to ensure that sex is safe and enjoyable. Having access to information about safe sex will give you the confidence to explore and fulfill your sexual desires with less anxiety. Ensuring that you are engaging in safe sex is a loving thing to do—for yourself and your partner.

Understanding the different types of sex and ways to make it safer is the first step in taking charge of your sexual health. Your sexual health is an important part of your overall health, and it includes discovering your sexual identity and attractions, finding ways to communicate them to others, and preventing the transmission of STIs.

This section breaks down the various acts of sexual intimacy in the following way:

- Penetrative sex

- Oral Sex

- Sex with hands

- Sex with toys

PENETRATIVE SEX

Penetrative sex is when someone inserts their genitals or another body part inside their partner's front hole, vagina, mouth, or anus. It is also sometimes called *intercourse*. The person being penetrated, the "bottom," has a higher risk for contracting STIs than the one who's doing the penetrating, the "top."

To make penetrative sex safer, always use a barrier like a condom or dental dam. Most are made out of latex, but if you have a latex allergy, you can find ones made of polyisoprene or polyurethane. Make sure you put it on correctly and that you use a new barrier with each new sexual partner and activity.

Never put more than one condom on a penis at one time. Using two condoms on the same penis increases friction, which increases the chance that one or both condoms will break.

Also, apply lube liberally. Lube cuts down on the amount of friction on a condom, which helps prevent the chance that the condom will break. It can also be helpful to place lube on the front hole, vagina, or anus before insertion. Lube can decrease pain and friction while increasing pleasure.

ORAL SEX

Oral sex is when someone uses their mouth, tongue, throat, and even teeth to stimulate a partner's genitals (clitoris, front hole, vagina, penis, or scrotum) or anus. To make oral sex safer, place a barrier (e.g., a dental dam or condom) between the mouth and body part receiving oral sex.

SAFE-SEX BASICS

If you're sexually active, get tested often for STIs and talk with your partners about the last time they were tested. Check out gettested. cdc.gov to find a clinic near you, or visit www.stdtestexpress.com if you need an at-home STI test kit. Because some STIs don't come with significant or visible symptoms, many people with an STI do not know they have one.

Always use barriers, for example, male or female condoms, gloves, and dental dams, and apply lube.

Don't engage in sex (especially oral or penetrative) if you notice cuts, sores, bumps, or high-risk bodily fluids (blood) on your partner's genitals or in their mouth because this can be a sign of an infection and increase the chances of transmitting an STI.

SEX WITH HANDS

You can use your fingers and hands during sex to stimulate parts of the body, for instance, the penis, front hole, anus, vagina, mouth, or nipples. Wash your hands and clip your fingernails beforehand. When touching your partner, use a hand or glove that's different from the one you use to touch yourself. Although sex with hands and fingers isn't a common way of transmitting STIs, it can still happen.

SEX WITH TOYS

Sex toys are great for solo use (masturbation) or sex with your partner. Sex toys include vibrators (can be used on the front hole and vagina), dildos (can be used on the front hole, vagina, and anus), plugs (can be used anally), and beads (can be used anally). These toys help stimulate body parts internally and externally.

When you're with a partner, you should still use protection when using toys. Viruses and bacteria can spread from inanimate objects like vibrators. Use a condom on toys used for penetration in the front hole, vagina, anus, or mouth. If your toy was exposed to such bodily fluids as semen, vaginal fluids, saliva, or blood, try not to share it to reduce the risk of transmitting an STI.

If you do decide to share a sex toy that was used by or with a previous partner, clean it thoroughly, following the manufacturer's instructions. Depending on the material they are made of, some should be cleaned using soap and water, while others should be boiled in water. Make sure you follow the manufacturer's instructions.

SAFE SEX IS NOT BORING SEX

The opposite is true. Practicing safe sex will give you the comfort and confidence to explore and fulfill your sexual desires with less anxiety. When you know you can trust your partner and are free from worries about STIs, you can more fully explore your sexuality and enjoy your experiences.

ALL ABOUT STIs

Did you know that one in two sexually active people will contract an STI (sexually transmitted infection—an infection that's passed from one person to another through sexual contact and activity) by age twenty-five in the United States, and many don't even know they have an STI?[4] Although there's often a lot of negative stigma concerning contracting STIs, it's a common occurrence. The good news is that most STIs can be treated with medication, and many can be cured with antibiotics. If you ignore the risk factors and don't treat your STI, serious health issues can result.

There are many ways that STIs can be transmitted.

- Skin-to-skin contact

- Vaginal/front hole sex

- Anal sex

- Oral sex

- Contact with bodily fluids, for example, blood or semen

- Needles

You cannot get STIs from drinking out of someone else's glass, someone sneezing on you, the water fountain, or other casual contacts. Kissing results in a very, very low risk for herpes and syphilis. If you see open sores on someone's mouth, it is best not to kiss them until they heal. It's rare for STIs to spread via kissing, but it can happen.

Some of the most common STIs include the following:

- Gonorrhea (bacterial): Left untreated, can lead to infertility.

- Chlamydia (bacterial): Left untreated, can lead to infertility.

- Syphilis (bacterial): Left untreated, can lead to brain damage or death.

- Human papillomavirus (HPV) (viral): Left untreated, can lead to cancer.

- Herpes (viral): Left untreated, can lead to recurring sores and higher rates of transmission.

- HIV (viral): Left untreated, can lead to death.

- Hepatitis C (viral): Left untreated, can lead to cancer or death.

If you have a bacterial STI, you'll need to take a course of antibiotics. Most viral STIs, on the other hand, can't be cured with antibiotics. The only one that can be entirely cured with treatment in most cases is hepatitis C. There are also vaccinations for hepatitis C and HPV, which prevent you from getting the virus. They don't treat or cure it if you already have it.

If you become infected with a viral STI (other than hepatitis C), you'll always be a carrier of that virus. Medications help decrease the chances of transmission and protect you against serious health issues, but they can't eradicate the virus inside the body.

When they properly use medications and practice safe sex, most people with viral STIs can effectively manage symptoms and reduce their risk of transmitting the infection to their partners. If you are a carrier for any viral STI, you need to be honest with all your sexual partners and tell them before you engage in any sexual acts. Barriers like condoms and dental dams will protect your partners, but they still have the right to know and decide for themselves.

As you learned earlier in the chapter, there are effective ways to prevent getting an STI while still enjoying a fulfilling sex life. They are as follows:

- Frequent STI testing (at least once a year)

- Condoms, dental dams, and gloves used correctly with each sex act

- Medications like preexposure prophylaxis (PrEP) or postexposure prophylaxis (PEP)

- Vaccinations

Talking with your healthcare provider about these options can help you decide which combination of methods makes the most sense for your situation. If you don't have an LGBTQIA+-supportive healthcare provider you can confide in, try the local Planned Parenthood (www.plannedparenthood.org).

GETTING AND GIVING CONSENT

Sexual consent is the act of agreeing to participate in touching or other sexual encounters. Consent should be part of every sexual activity you engage in, including every type of touching. That includes kissing.

When there are multiple stages to your sexual interaction, you need to get consent—and consent to each phase. Consenting to one stage doesn't mean someone is consenting to every stage. Also, it's important to remember that the absence of a "no" does not imply a "yes."

Consent is usually more than just a simple yes or no. Check in with your sexual partner before and during sexual behaviors to help create a safe environment. Then your sexual experiences can be mutually pleasurable and positive, and based on respect and understanding. Take time *beforehand* to talk about consent and sex, as well as barriers and protections. Talking beforehand allows you to stay in the moment while being clear about what's okay and what isn't.

Consent is an important and serious aspect of sex, but it doesn't have to be a mood-killer. There are lots of ways to give and receive consent. When you find the ones that work for you, it can help create trust and open communication. The main takeaway is to talk about consent before things get steamy.

> *Having a crush on someone who was so open and free with*
> *her sexuality, and who seemed to accept me just as I was,*
> *helped me come to terms with being gay. It was like she was*
> *an example of how I wanted to live in the world. Before I*
> *met her, I didn't even realize it was possible to be that free.*
> —Stephanie, identifies as lesbian, age nineteen

ARE YOU READY?

You may feel that your relationship is ready when you can be completely honest and trust the other person, and the other person can trust you. Can you talk to your partner about such topics as past relationships, feelings, STIs, and sexual desires? Do you feel free to protect yourself and your partner against STIs? Do you respect the other person's decisions and sexual boundaries, and do they respect yours?

If you are in love or like someone, it's sometimes hard to see the signs of an unhealthy relationship. If your partner is overly jealous or possessive, manipulates you by bullying you or threatening to hurt themself or you if you end the relationship, or pressures you to have sex and refuses to see your point of view, it's not a good idea to engage in sex with that person. Refer back to the section at the beginning of this chapter titled "Signs of an Unhealthy Relationship" for more information about healthy relationships.

SEX SHOULD NEVER BE FORCED

No one should ever be forced to have sex. If you are ever forced to have sex, never blame yourself, and tell an adult you trust as soon as possible.

Only you can decide when it's time. If your partner is pressuring you or intimidating you, take it as a warning—this person does not have your best interests at heart.

MAKING IT GOOD

If you think you might be ready for your first sexual experience, consider these tips to help make it the best it can be.

- *Do it with someone you love, someone who cares for you, and someone who respects you.* It will be much harder to regret and less likely take a toll on your self-esteem if you care about the person and they care about you.

- *Don't expect it to be like porn, and don't use porn as your guide.* Porn is not real, and it will more than likely make you a selfish lover, or at least a misguided one.

- *Talk to your partner ahead of time about expectations, desires, and, of course, consent.* Talking about what you need and listening to what they need can be a real turn-on and will greatly increase the chances of you both being satisfied.

- *Keep your expectations low.* It's your first time. It might not be great. Make the mood enticing (music, candles, lighting, lube, etc.), and try to enjoy the process. You'll become a better lover throughout time if you listen to what your partner wants and needs. Don't be afraid to ask for what you need.

- *Don't forget the foreplay.* Just because you've agreed that tonight is the big night doesn't mean you should jump right into the act. Take your time and build up to it, with whatever means you both enjoy— kissing, touching, hand stimulation, oral sex, toys, and so on.

- *Don't fake it.* Faking it the first time only sets a precedent for you to keep on faking it. Show your partner how to pleasure you instead.

- *Use lube!* It adds to the pleasure and sensation, and it helps prevent friction-related sores and pain.

- *Always use protection.* Set the pattern in your relationship right away. It protects you both. You might feel weird or uncomfortable mentioning this at first, but as it becomes the norm, you'll be really glad you did. If you have a partner who fights the use of protection, that's a red flag. Educate them on the risks. See the section on STIs for more information.

MAKE SOBER CHOICES

If you've been using alcohol or drugs, you're not in a good state to make important decisions about sex. Too many young people have sex without meaning to (or without protection) when they drink alcohol or use drugs.

GRACE'S BEST MOMENT

Grace struggled with her sexuality for a long time. She knew she wasn't quite straight but also felt she wasn't fully a lesbian. What was she? Like many people, she thought that being bisexual was just a label for people who couldn't decide or couldn't accept they were gay.

This struggle followed her into college. She had dated very little at that point, one or two guys, very briefly. But the confusing feelings continued.

One day during her sophomore year, a girl who lived in her dorm, who Grace knew was gay, asked Grace to go with her to a Gay Pride rally that was happening on campus. Grace's first thought was, "Why would she ask me to go—do I seem gay to her?" Something inside convinced her to say yes, even though the idea of it scared her to death.

She'll never forget walking through the buildings to the quad area where the rally was being held. The scene opened up to her like a beautiful field of daisies, all different colors. People of different orientations and gender identities were holding signs and mulling together, celebrating. They seemed so comfortable and proud to be in their own skin. They were there to celebrate who they were. It was so beautiful and revolutionary, and normal, at the same time. Grace was overcome with emotions—feelings of happiness, but also sadness. She felt sad about how she had been treating herself. How could she have been so unkind to herself all this time?

That day, she took her first steps toward accepting herself. No matter where that path led, she would accept herself and be okay with it. The amazing community she saw that day inspired her and gave her the courage she didn't think she had.

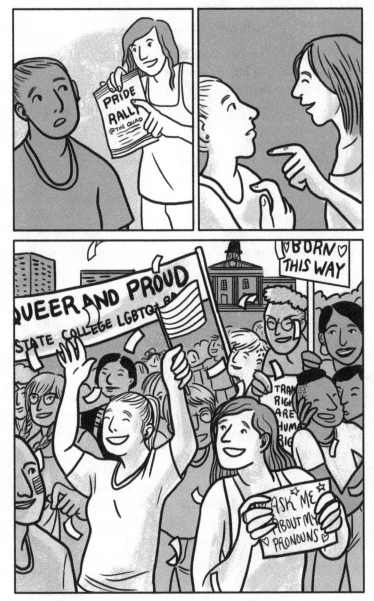

Grace was struggling with her sexuality when a college friend asked
her to go to a Gay Pride rally, which inspired her to be kinder to herself.
Illustration by Kate Haberer

The first sexual experience is special. You and your partner may not have amazing orgasms this first go-around, but you should still get pleasure from the experience. Take the time to figure out what's going to satisfy you and your partner both physically and mentally during your first time.

THE JOURNEY TO A FULFILLING QUEER LIFE

All close relationships need attention, work, and patience. That goes for teen relationships, too, regardless of your orientation. The most important and longest-lasting relationship you'll have in your life is the one you have with *you*. Get right with you before you bring a loved one on board. Treat yourself with love and kindness—only then can you treat others the same way.

> *This might sound corny, but I do really believe that the power of love can change even the most stubborn minds. I've seen it in my own life. It may not happen overnight, but it can happen.*
> —Grant, identifies as gay, age twenty-two

Relationships, intimacy, and sex are wonderful parts of the human experience. If you're not ready for them, they can also be very hurtful and damaging to your self-esteem. Take your time and trust yourself to know what you need, and only *you* get to decide when.

CHAPTER SEVEN

LIVING HAPPY AND GAY

Being gay is like glitter; it never goes away.
—Lady Gaga

SEEKING A BETTER UNDERSTANDING

It might sound cliché, but to be truly happy, we all need to learn to love and accept ourselves. For someone who identifies as LGBTQIA+ in our homophobic society, that can be a particularly difficult process.

Studies have shown that rates of depression and emotional instability in gay men who are "out" are not higher than averages for heterosexual men.[1] Moreover, less internalized homophobia in LGBTQIA+ adults was connected with fewer thoughts of suicide and less overall loneliness.[2] That is good news. When you come out at your own pace, come to terms with who you are (the good and the "bad"), and work on loving and accepting yourself, you can have a fulfilling and happy life ahead of you.

This chapter discusses various issues that you may run into as you work toward becoming a healthy, happy, self-fulfilled, contributing member of society.

BENEFITS OF BEING QUEER

Aside from the most obvious benefit of being yourself rather than hurtfully hiding who you are, did you know that there are advantages to being queer, as reported consistently by LGBTQIA+ adults? Consider these perks:

- You are likely to become more empathetic and compassionate toward anyone who is discriminated against for any reason.

- You may feel more freed from social constraints related to gender roles and expectations in relationships. For example, you may feel more ownership in deciding your role in a relationship, regardless of gender. You can more easily reject gender traditions and stereotypes that you don't like or don't fit your persona.

- You have access to a community of friends who are more likely to be loyal and understanding.

- You may find that you develop better relationships with heterosexuals throughout time. With the gender norms and sexual expectations out of the way, you can be a nonthreatening friend to same-sex or different-sex heterosexuals.[3]

Every gay and lesbian person who has been lucky enough to survive the turmoil of growing up is a survivor. Survivors always have an obligation to those who will face the same challenges.
—Bob Paris, writer and actor

You live in a time in which, in most towns and cities in the United States at least, LGBTQIA+ people no longer have to suffer invisibility. They are out and will stay out. In the larger legal society, LGBTQIA+ people have the freedom to be themselves and love whoever they want, regardless of gender. Things can certainly be better—in churches, in workplaces, in small towns, and elsewhere—but there's reason to celebrate where we are now.

BUILD FRIENDSHIPS YOU CAN COUNT ON

Like all relationships, good friendships have to be created, nurtured, developed, and maintained by both parties. They aren't self-driving machines. If you want gay friends, it makes sense to go where gay people may hang out, for example, at a GSA meeting, a LGBTQIA+ community center meeting, or a Pride celebration.

WHEN MICHAEL FOUND HIS TRIBE

Michael had been out, "casually" as he calls it, for some time by the time he turned sixteen. His close friends knew, and he was starting to think his parents had some idea and were not entirely scared away by the idea. He hadn't talked to them directly about it and was terrified to do so, but he also had had a few boyfriends and lived his online life "out and proud."

What he wanted was to connect to a LGBTQIA+ group. Even though his friends were somewhat supportive and his parents hadn't thrown him out (yet), he still felt alienated and alone. His New Year's resolution that year was to find connections with the broader LGBTQIA+ community.

After searching for a while in his hometown, Michael became discouraged. If groups were out there, they were hard to find. His high school did not have a LGBTQIA+ support group, so, after lots of consideration and fear and worries, he decided to start one. In the first meeting, two people came. The three of them just sat in the classroom and exchanged stories for an hour. In the next meeting, four people came. Some were straight and wanted to be allies for the LGBTQIA+ teens in their high school. They changed the name of the club to the Gay–Straight Alliance (GSA), and more people joined. During the next school year, Michael became the unofficial president of this club, and they set about educating the student body about body image issues, LGBTQIA+ role models, gender identity, overcoming isolation, and more.

The club became a fixture at the school that many students talked and knew about. They even raised the most money while fundraising two years in a row. The best part for Michael was that he created a community from his need for connection, and it helped lots of people with theirs. It gave him the confidence to live his life fully, on his terms.

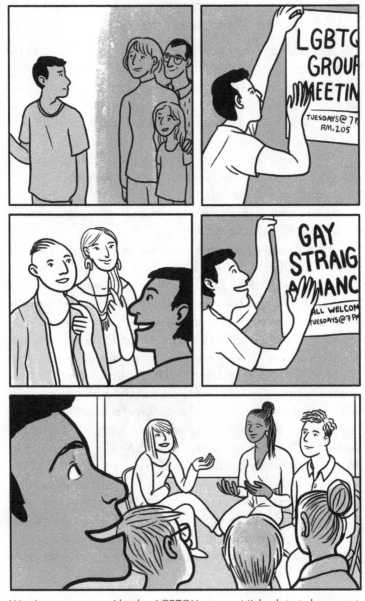

Wanting to connect with other LGBTQIA+ teens, Michael started a support group at his school. *Illustration by Kate Haberer*

A Pride celebration is an annual event that commemorates the beginning of gay liberation. Cities usually have a parade and festival that occur in June. Pride is an excellent time to meet other gay and lesbian folks in a fun and celebratory atmosphere. Consider marching in the Pride parade or attending a Pride concert or event. These are activities that could lead to new friendships and connections. LGBTQIA+ Pride celebrations have a wide variety of activities associated with them. There is usually a parade, but there are also often concerts, parties, and festivals.

Also, consider volunteering for a gay or lesbian organization. You are sure to meet other gays and lesbians if you volunteer for an organization that is working for gay rights. Pick an organization that is fighting for a cause in which you believe. That way, you will make a difference in the world, and you may make some good friends at the same time.

You can get involved in a wide variety of causes. For instance, organizations are working for the legal rights of LGBTQIA+ folks to end violence, discrimination, and teen homelessness, and a ton of other causes. Pick the cause that is most important to you.

QueerBFF is a networking app that helps you find platonic friendships with other LGBTQIA+ people and connect with LGBTQIA+ wherever you are at the moment. You can find it on the Apple Store or Google Store online. Before you download an app like this, be sure to read the section in this chapter about staying safe online.

Whatever ways you seek out friendships, make an active point of spending your time with positive, supportive people. Spending time with positive people can help you be more positive in your own life. Other people's attitudes are contagious. Focus on the blessings in your life and take time to feel gratitude for people or things that are going well and supporting you right now.

PITFALLS TO AVOID

Beyond the good news, there are dangers out there for all young people who are navigating the world, and that is often even truer for LGBTQIA+ young people. This section discusses some of the issues that plague the LGBTQIA+ community in larger numbers.

I didn't want to come out to my parents until I felt like I'd come
to terms with being a lesbian. I'd had a few girlfriends already.
The relationship I had at the time was starting to feel serious.
So I thought it was time for them to know. I was tired of hiding
everything. When I told my parents about my girlfriend, they were
really supportive. They asked when they could meet her. It was still
awkward for a long while, but I appreciated that they were trying.
                    —Jenn, identifies as gay, age twenty-three

MENTAL HEALTH ISSUES

Multiple studies have shown that LGBTQIA+ youth tend to suffer higher rates of depression, anxiety, and suicidal ideation (thoughts) than other teen groups. For example, the Human Rights Campaign's "2018 LGBTQ Youth Report" found that 77 percent of LGBTQIA+ youth surveyed reported that, on average, they had felt down or depressed in the past week. Only 41 percent had received psychological or emotional counseling in the past year. LGBTQIA+ youth of color have even greater challenges in accessing counseling services, with large differences and an average of 37 percent having received psychological or emotional counseling in the past year. Youth who had received culturally competent, LGBTQIA-affirming counseling reported better mental health outcomes.[4]

How do you know if you're dealing with a level of depression or anxiety that you need to address? According to *Psychology Today*, two simple questions can help recognize depression: (1) During the past month, have you often been bothered by feeling down, depressed, or hopeless? and (2) During the past month, have you often been bothered by little interest or pleasure in doing things?[5] If you answered "yes" to these questions, it's time to make some lifestyle changes and seek support.

It's important to realize that these increased issues with depression and anxiety are not because you are queer, so you must be "mentally ill," no matter what you've heard in the world around you, but because you face greater threats of violence and stigma, could be bullied or made fun of, are not accepted by friends or family, and may feel alone in your journey to self-acceptance. People in general—teens and adults, gay and straight—who feel isolated, unaccepted, and alone report higher levels of depression and anxiety across the board.[6] If you feel this way, it's not because you are inherently bad, but because you aren't getting the support and acceptance that we all need as human beings. Psychologists have given this a name—"minority stress"—and it suggests that people who feel left out of a group are better off if they join forces with others like them than if they try to cope on their own.[7]

SEEK HELP

LGBTQIA+ youth who come from highly rejecting families are 8.4 times as likely to have attempted suicide as LGBTQIA+ peers who reported no or low levels of family rejection.[8] If your family has rejected you, be aware of feelings of worthlessness, practice self-care and self-love, and seek help dealing with these feelings of rejection.

As we have said and as you no doubt know, we can't control other people's reactions to us. So what can you do to ease the burden of being a LGBTQIA+ teen in your community?

The National Suicide Prevention Lifeline number is 1-800-273-8255. Reach out for help. There are many people out there who understand what you're going through and want to help.

Ideas to help navigate the world of depression and mental health are the same coping skills we've been discussing throughout the book.

- *Come out to supportive people.* Remember that being out usually brings more positive outcomes, including better academic performance, higher self-esteem, and lower anxiety and depression.[9] Of course, you need to consider your safety and other issues as you decide who to tell. If you can find even one supportive person or group (even online) you can positively come out to, that can help a lot.

- *Seek culturally competent, LGBTQIA-affirming counseling.* The key here is that it needs to be "culturally competent and LGBTQIA-affirming." No "gay conversion" therapy for you. For one, it has shown time and again not to work.[10] More importantly, there is nothing wrong with who you are—you don't need to be converted or fixed. If you can't find local support, check out www.thetrevor-project.org online.

- *Find support groups.* Many support groups are referenced throughout this book and in the "Resources" section. Joining a group of like-minded people, especially when you come together for a larger cause, can fill you with hope, connectedness, and purposefulness.

- *Practice self-care through lifestyle changes.* In addition to making connections and getting counseling, simple changes like regular exercise, getting enough sunlight, and developing better sleeping habits have been effective in treating depression.

- *Consider antidepressant medication.* The evidence as to whether such antidepressants as SSRIs (selective serotonin reuptake inhibitors like Prozac and Zoloft) help or hurt adolescents and teens is conflicting. For some, they can significantly improve mood, help with anxiety, and diminish sleep disorders. For others, they can increase suicidal thoughts and cause mood disorders to worsen. The Food and Drug Administration has issued a "black box" warning for all antidepressants in young people up to the age of twenty-four because of the

NOTES

YOU ARE NOT ALONE

1. Centers for Disease Control and Prevention, National Center for Injury Prevention and Control, "Web-Based Injury Statistics Query and Reporting System (WISQARS)," last modified 2019, https://webapp .cdc.gov/cgi-bin/broker.exe.
2. Centers for Disease Control and Prevention, *Sexual Identity, Sex of Sexual Contacts, and Health-Risk Behaviors among Students in Grades 9–12: Youth Risk Behaviour Surveillance* (Atlanta, GA: U.S. Department of Health and Human Services, 2019).
3. Human Rights Campaign, "Growing Up LGBT in America: View and Share Statistics," last modified 2020, https://www.hrc.org/youth-re port/view-and-share-statistics.
4. Human Rights Campaign, "Growing Up LGBT in America: About the Survey," last modified 2020, https://www.hrc.org/youth-report/about -the-survey.
5. Pew Research Center, "Support Steady for Same-Sex Marriage and Acceptance of Homosexuality," last modified May 12, 2016, https://www.pewresearch.org/fact-tank/2016/05/12/support-steady -for-same-sex-marriage-and-acceptance-of-homosexuality/.
6. Pew Research Center, "A Survey of LGBT Americans," last modified June 13, 2013, https://www.pewsocialtrends.org/2013/06/13/a-survey -of-lgbt-americans/.
7. Gallup, "Gay and Lesbian Rights," last modified 2020, https://news .gallup.com/poll/1651/gay-lesbian-rights.aspx.

8. Pew Research Center, "Chapter 3: The Coming Out Experience," last modified June 13, 2013, https://www.pewsocialtrends.org/2013/06/13/chapter-3-the-coming-out-experience/#fn-17196-14.

CHAPTER ONE: UNDERSTANDING YOUR SEXUALITY AND PERSONAL IDENTITY

1. Human Rights Campaign, "Sexual Orientation and Gender Identity Definitions," last modified 2020, https://www.hrc.org/resources/sexual-orientation-and-gender-identity-terminology-and-definitions.
2. Ritch C. Savin-Williams and Kenneth M. Cohen, "Mostly Straight, Most of the Time," *Good Men Project*, September 18, 2018, https://goodmenproject.com/featured-content/mostly-straight/.
3. Lisa M. Diamond, *Sexual Fluidity: Understanding Women's Love and Desire* (Cambridge, MA: Harvard University Press, 2008).
4. Richard H. Reams, "A Guide for People Who Question Their Sexual Orientation: Part 3: Myths," *Your Sexual Orientation*, https://yoursexualorientation.info/myths.
5. Trevor Project, "Coming Out: A Handbook for LGBTQ Young People," last modified October 2019, https://www.thetrevorproject.org/wp-content/uploads/2019/10/Coming-Out-Handbook.pdf.

CHAPTER TWO: DEALING WITH NEGATIVE FEELINGS AND BUILDING SELF-RESPECT

1. Centers for Disease Control and Prevention, *Sexual Identity, Sex of Sexual Contacts, and Health-Risk Behaviors among Students in Grades 9–12: Youth Risk Behavior Surveillance* (Atlanta, GA: U.S. Department of Health and Human Services, 2019).
2. Human Rights Campaign, "Growing Up LGBT in America," last modified 2020, https://www.hrc.org/youth-report/view-and-share-statistics.
3. Human Rights Campaign. "Growing Up LGBT in America."
4. D. M. Barnes and I. Meyer, "Religious Affiliation, Internalized Homophobia, and Mental Health in Lesbians, Gay Men, and Bisexuals," *American Journal of Orthopsychiatry* 82, no. 4 (2012): 505–15.

5. K. Kralovec, C. Fartacek, R. Fartacek, and M. Plöderl, "Religion and Suicide Risk in Lesbian, Gay, and Bisexual Australians," *Journal of Religion and Health* 53, no. 2 (April 2014): 413–23.

6. Mychal Copeland, "It's Time to Rethink Religion vs. LGBT," *Huffpost*, February 26, 2017, https://www.huffpost.com/entry/its-time-to-rethink-religion-v-lgbt_b_9301566.

7. Pew Research Center, "A Survey of LGBT Americans," last modified June 13, 2013, https://www.pewsocialtrends.org/2013/06/13/a-survey-of-lgbt-americans/.

8. Stephanie Pappas, "Five Surprising Facts about Gay Conversion Therapy," *LiveScience*, June 43, 2013, https://www.livescience.com/37139-facts-about-gay-conversion-therapy.html.

9. Emily Reynolds, "The Cruel, Dangerous Reality of Gay Conversion Therapy," *Wired*, July 7, 2018, https://www.wired.co.uk/article/what-is-gay-conversion-therapy.

10. American Psychological Association, *Report of the American Psychological Association Task Force on Appropriate Therapeutic Responses to Sexual Orientation*, last modified 2019, https://www.apa.org/pi/lgbt/resources/therapeutic-response.pdf.

11. American Academy of Child and Adolescent Psychiatry, "Conversion Therapy," last modified February 2018, https://www.aacap.org/aacap/policy_statements/2018/Conversion_Therapy.aspx.

12. Human Rights Campaign, "Policy and Position Statements on Conversion Therapy," last modified 2020, https://www.hrc.org/resources/policy-and-position-statements-on-conversion-therapy.

13. Centers for Disease Control and Prevention, "LGBT Youth," last modified June 21, 2017, https://www.cdc.gov/lgbthealth/youth.htm.

14. Darrell C. Greene and Paula J. Britton, "The Influence of Forgiveness on Lesbian, Gay, Bisexual, Transgender, and Questioning Individuals' Shame and Self-Esteem," *Journal of Counseling and Development* 91, no. 2 (2013): 195–205.

15. Greene and Britton, "The Influence of Forgiveness on Lesbian, Gay, Bisexual, Transgender, and Questioning Individuals' Shame and Self-Esteem."

16. Tom Bruett, "Ways for Gay Men to Improve Self-Esteem," *Tom Bruett Therapy*, February 25, 2019, https://tombruetttherapy.com/improve-your-self-esteem-as-a-gay-man/.

CHAPTER THREE: ARE YOU READY TO COME OUT?

1. Anne Dohrenwend, *Coming Around: Parenting Lesbian, Gay, Bisexual, and Transgender Kids* (Far Hills, NJ: New Horizon Press, 2012).
2. The Trevor Project, "Coming Out: A Handbook for LGBTQ Young People," last modified 2020, https://www.thetrevorproject.org/trvr_support_center/coming-out/.
3. Michael C. LaSala, "Gay Male Couples: The Importance of Coming Out and Being Out to Parents," *Journal of Homosexuality* 39, no. 2 (2000): 47–71; Lewis et al., "An Empirical Analysis of Stressors for Gay Men and Lesbians," *Journal of Homosexuality* 43, no. 1 (2001): 63–88; S. A. Halpin and M. W. Allen, "Changes in Psychological Well-Being during Stages of Gay Identity Development," *Journal of Homosexuality* 47, no. 1 (2004): 109–26; Richard Allen Stevens, "Understanding Gay Identity Development within the College Environment," *Journal of College Student Development* 45, no. 2 (2004): 185–206.
4. S. W. Cole, M. E. Kemeny, and S. E. Taylor, "Elevated Physical Health Risk among Gay Men Who Conceal Their Sexual Identity," *Health Psychology* 15, no. 4 (July 1996): 243–51; Belle Rose Ragins, Romila Singh, and John M. Cornwell, "Making the Invisible Visible: Fear and Disclosure of Sexual Orientation at Work," *Journal of Applied Psychology* 92, no. 4 (August 2007): 1103–18.
5. Human Rights Campaign, "Growing Up LGBT in America," last modified 2020, https://www.hrc.org/youth-report/view-and-share-statistics.
6. F. J. Floyd and R. Bakeman, "Coming Out across the Life Course: Implications of Age and Historical Context," *Archives of Sexual Behavior* 35 (2006): 287–96.
7. N. B. Doty, B. L. B. Willoughby, K. M. Lindahl, and N. M. Malik, "Sexuality Related Social Support among Lesbian, Gay, and Bisexual Youth," *Journal of Youth and Adolescence* 39, no. 10 (2010): 1134–47.
8. Laurie Heatherington and Justin Lavner, "Coming to Terms with Coming Out: Review and Recommendations for Family-Systems Focused Research," *Journal of Family Psychology* 22, no. 3 (2008): 329–43.
9. V. Cass, "Homosexual Identity Formation: A Theoretical Model," *Journal of Homosexuality* 4, no. 3 (1979): 219–35.

CHAPTER FOUR: DEALING WITH REACTIONS

1. "Heteronormative," *Merriam-Webster*, https://www.merriam-webster .com/dictionary/heteronormative.
2. American Psychological Association, "Lesbian, Gay, Bisexual, and Transgender Aging," last modified 2020, https://www.apa.org/pi/lgbt/ resources/aging.
3. K. Kralovec, C. Fartacek, R. Fartacek, and M. Plöderl, "Religion and Suicide Risk in Lesbian, Gay, and Bisexual Australians," *Journal of Religion and Health* 53, no. 2 (April 2014): 413–23.
4. Anne Dohrenwend, *Coming Around: Parenting Gay, Bisexual, and Transgender Kids* (Far Hills, NJ: New Horizon Press, 2012), 60.
5. Human Rights Campaign, "2018 LGBTQ Youth Report," last modified 2020, https://www.hrc.org/resources/2018-lgbtq-youth-report.
6. Human Rights Campaign, "2018 LGBTQ Youth Report."
7. Human Rights Campaign, "2018 LGBTQ Youth Report."
8. Centers for Disease Control and Prevention, "Lesbian, Gay, Bisexual, and Transgender Health," last modified 2020, https://www.cdc.gov/ lgbthealth/youth.htm.
9. Urban Institute, "Teen Dating Abuse in the Digital Age," last modified 2020, https://www.urban.org/features/teen-dating-abuse-digital-age.
10. Centers for Disease Control and Prevention, "Gay and Bisexual Men's Health," last modified 2020, https://www.cdc.gov/msmhealth/stigma -and-discrimination.htm.

CHAPTER FIVE: BUILDING A SUPPORT NETWORK

1. Centers for Disease Control and Prevention, "Lesbian, Gay, Bisexual, and Transgender Health: Youth Resources," last modified 2020, https:// www.cdc.gov/lgbthealth/youth-resources.htm.
2. R. B. Toomey, C. Ryan, R. M. Diaz, and S. T. Russell, "High School Gay–Straight Alliances (GSAs) and Young Adult Well-Being: An Examination of GSA Presence, Participation, and Perceived Effectiveness," *Applied Developmental Science* 15, no. 4 (2011): 175–85.
3. Toomey, Ryan, Diaz, and Russell, "High School Gay–Straight Alliances (GSAs) and Young Adult Well-Being."

4. Gay, Lesbian, and Straight Education Network, "Ten Steps to Start Your GSA," last modified 2020, https://www.glsen.org/sites/default/files/2019-11/GLSEN-10-Steps-To-Start-Your-GSA.pdf.

5. Daniel Greenberg, Emma Beyer, Maxine Najle, Oyindamola Bola, and Robert P. Jones, "Americans Show Broad Support for LGBT Nondiscrimination Protections," *Public Religion Research Institute*, last modified March 12, 2019, https://www.prri.org/research/americans-support-protections-lgbt-people/.

6. Pew Research Center, "A Survey of LGBT Americans," last modified June 13, 2013, https://www.pewsocialtrends.org/2013/06/13/a-survey-of-lgbt-americans/.

CHAPTER SIX: SEX AND LOVE

1. Laura Kann, Tim McManus, and William A. Harris, "Youth Risk Behavior Surveillance—United States, 2017," *Morbidity and Mortality Weekly Report* 67, no. 8 (2018): 1–114, https://www.cdc.gov/mmwr/volumes/67/ss/ss6708a1.htm.

2. Urban Institute, "Teen Dating Abuse in the Digital Age," last modified 2020, https://www.urban.org/features/teen-dating-abuse-digital-age.

3. Gay, Lesbian, and Straight Education Network, "2015 National School Climate Survey," last modified 2019, https://www.glsen.org/research/2015-national-school-climate-survey.

4. J. R. Cates, N. L. Herndon, S. L. Schulz, and J. E. Darroch, *Our Voices, Our Lives, Our Futures: Youth and Sexually Transmitted Diseases* (Chapel Hill: University of North Carolina at Chapel Hill School of Journalism and Mass Communication, 2004), http://joancates.web.unc.edu/files/2010/11/Our-Voices-Our-Lives-Our-Futures-Youth-and-Sexually-Transmitted-Diseases.pdf.

CHAPTER SEVEN: LIVING HAPPY AND GAY

1. Jane A. Bybee, Eric L. Sullivan, Erich Zielonka, and Elizabeth Moes, "Are Gay Men in Worse Mental Health Than Heterosexual Men? The

Role of Age, Shame, and Guilt, and Coming Out," *Journal of Adult Development* 16, no. 3 (2009): 144–54.

2. Anthony R. D'Augelli and Arnold H. Grossman, "Disclosure of Sexual Orientation, Victimization, and Mental Health among Lesbian, Gay, and Bisexual Older Adults," *Journal of Interpersonal Violence* 16, no. 10 (October 2001): 1,008–27.

3. Riggle, Ellen D. B., Joy S. Whitman, Amber Olson, Sharon Scales Rostosky, and Sue Strong. "The Positive Aspects of Being a Lesbian or Gay Man." *Professional Psychology: Research and Practice* 39 no. 2 (2008): 210–217.

4. Human Rights Campaign, "2018 LGBTQ Youth Report," last modified 2020, https://www.hrc.org/resources/2018-lgbtq-youth-report.

5. John-Manuel Andriote, "Depression Is Killing Gay Men," *Psychology Today*, June 14, 2018, https://www.psychologytoday.com/us/blog/stonewall-strong/201806/depression-is-killing-gay-men.

6. Amy Novotney, "Social Isolation: It Could Kill You," *American Psychological Association* 50, no. 5 (May 2019), https://www.apa.org/monitor/2019/05/ce-corner-isolation.

7. Michael P. Dentato, "The Minority Stress Perspective," *American Psychological Association Psychology and AIDS Exchange Newsletter*, April 2002, https://www.apa.org/pi/aids/resources/exchange/2012/04/minority-stress.

8. C. Ryan, D. Huebner, R. M. Diaz, and J. Sanchez, "Family Rejection as a Predictor of Negative Health Outcomes in White and Latino Lesbian, Gay, and Bisexual Young Adults," *Pediatrics* 123, no. 1 (January 2009): 346–52.

9. Stephen T. Russell and Jessica N. Fish, "Mental Health in Lesbian, Gay, Bisexual, and Transgender (LGBT) Youth," *Annual Review of Clinical Psychology* 12 (March 2016): 465–87.

10. Human Rights Campaign, "The Lies and Dangers of Efforts to Change Sexual Orientation or Gender Identity," last modified 2020, https://www.hrc.org/resources/the-lies-and-dangers-of-reparative-therapy.

11. Jeanne Lenzer, "FDA Panel Urges 'Black Box' Warning for Antidepressants," *BMJ* 329, no. 7,468 (September 2004): 702.

12. Centers for Disease Control and Prevention, "Adolescent and School Health: Health Considerations for LGBTQ Youth," last modified

2020, https://www.cdc.gov/healthyyouth/disparities/health-consider ations-lgbtq-youth.htm.

13. Bryan N. Cochran, K. Michelle Peavy, and Jennifer S. Robohm, "Do Specialized Services Exist for LGBT Individuals Seeking Treatment for Substance Misuse? A Study of Available Treatment Programs," *Substance Use and Misuse* 42, no. 1 (2007): 161–76, https://www .tandfonline.com/doi/abs/10.1080/10826080601094207?journal Code=isum20.

14. Andy Marra, "Out Online: The Experiences of LGBT Youth on the Internet," *Gay, Lesbian, and Straight Education Network*, July 10, 2013, https://www.glsen.org/news/out-online-experiences-lgbt-youth-internet.

15. Stay Safe Online, "What LGBTQ Communities Should Know about Online Safety," last modified 2020, https://staysafeonline.org/ resource/lgbtq-communities-know-online-safety/.

16. Stay Safe Online, "What LGBT Communities Should Know about Online Safety," last modified 2020, https://staysafeonline.org/wp-con tent/uploads/2017/09/What-LGBT-Communities-Should-Know -About-Online-Safety.pdf.

RESOURCES

Are you looking for more information and advice about coming out? Or maybe you want to learn how to connect to the broader LGBTQIA+ community? Do you want to know more about other people's experiences with coming out and how they have handled it, the good and the bad? These resources will provide a next step in connecting to a loving community, coming to terms with your sexuality, and building up your self-worth.

BOOKS

Belge, Kathy, and Marke Bieschke. *Queer: The Ultimate LGBT Guide for Teens*, 2nd ed. San Francisco, CA: Zest Books, 2019.

Bianchi, Anna. *Becoming an Ally to the Gender-Expansive Child*. London: Jessica Kingsley, 2018.

Brison, Kevin. *Coming Out: I Think I'm Gay: The Ultimate Guide to Self-Acceptance, Coming Out, Building a Support System, and Loving Your New Life*. LCPublifish LLC, 2014.

Bronski, Micheal, Ann Pellegrini, and Micheal Amico. *You Can Tell Just by Looking, and 20 Other Myths about LGBT Life and People*. Boston: Beacon, 2013.

Deschamps, David, and Bennet Singer. *LGBTQ Stats: Lesbian, Gay, Bisexual, Transgender, and Queer People by the Numbers*. New York: New Press, 2017.

Field, Pete. *How to Be Gay and Happy: Live the Life You Were Born to Live and Feel Good about Yourself*. Burbank, CA: Rainbow Champions, 2016.

Khalaf, Riyadh. *Yay! You're Gay! Now What? A Gay Boy's Guide to Life.*
London: Quarto, 2019.

Levithan, David, and Billy Merrell, eds. *The Full Spectrum: A New Generation of Writing about Gay, Lesbian, Bisexual, Transgender, Questioning, and Other Identities.* New York: Knopf Books for Young Readers, 2006.

Nealy, Elijah C. *Transgender Children and Youth.* New York: W. W. Norton & Company, 2017.

Savage, Dan, and Terry Miller, eds. *It Gets Better: Coming Out, Overcoming Bullying, and Creating a Life Worth Living.* New York: Penguin, 2012.

Signorile, Michelangelo. *Outing Yourself: How to Come Out as Lesbian or Gay to Your Family, Friends, and Coworkers.* New York: Fireside, 1996.

WEBSITES AND SUPPORT GROUPS

The following list is in no way exhaustive, but it can help point you to some great, supportive resources and give you a start in finding what you need.

CRISIS INTERVENTION

If you are struggling, perhaps using drugs, engaging in other risky behaviors, or having depressive and suicidal thoughts, there is help out there. There are people who understand your specific struggles and want to help.

LGBT National Help Center
www.glbthotline.org/talkline.html
    The LGBT National Help Center has an anonymous helpline, called the LGBT National Youth Talkline, at 1-800-246-7743.

The Trevor Project
www.thetrevorproject.org

The Trevor Project is a national organization that provides crisis intervention and suicide prevention services to LGBTQIA+ people age twenty-five and younger. The organization has a crisis intervention Life-Line (1-866-488-7386), a TrevorChat for confidential online instant messaging with a Trevor counselor, and a TrevorText (text START to 678678) for confidential online text messaging with a Trevor counselor.

National Suicide Prevention Lifeline
suicidepreventionlifeline.org/help-yourself/youth/
The National Suicide Prevention Lifeline provides free and confidential support 24/7 for people in distress, information on prevention, and crisis resources for those in need. The number is 1-800-273-8255.

Break the Cycle
www.breakthecycle.org
At Break the Cycle, the goal is to inspire and support young people ages twelve to twenty-four in building healthy relationships and creating a culture without relationship abuse. You can call 1-866-331-9474, chat online, or text "loveis" to 22522 to speak to someone.

Love Is Respect
www.loveisrespect.org
This is a resource that empowers youth to prevent and end dating abuse. It is a project of the National Domestic Violence Hotline.

GETTING SUPPORT AND MAKING CONNECTIONS

This section lists websites where you can find comfort, community, information, and support. Many of these sites are discussed in this book.

The Trevor Project's Trevor Space
www.trevorspace.org
In addition to crisis intervention mentioned previously, the Trevor Space.org site calls itself an "affirming international community for

LGBTQIA+ young people ages thirteen to twenty-four." Join it to make connections with LGBTQIA+ youth throughout the world.

Human Rights Campaign (HRC)
www.hrc.org

This is the largest LGBTQIA+ advocacy group in the United States. HRC envisions a world where LGBTQIA+ people are ensured their fundamental equal rights and can be open, honest, and safe at home, at work, and in the community. Check out their latest report, called "Growing Up LGBT in America," at www.hrc.org/youth-report/view-and-share-statistics, or their "Resource Guide to Coming Out," at www.hrc.org/resources/resource-guide-to-coming-out.

National Center for Lesbian Rights
www.nclrights.org

The National Center for Lesbian Rights is committed to advancing lesbian, gay, bisexual, and transgender equality through litigation, legislation, policy, and public education.

Q Card Project
www.qcardproject.com

The Q Card is an easy-to-use communication tool to empower LGBTQIA+ youth to become actively engaged in their health and support the people who provide their care.

The Bisexual Resource Center
biresource.org

Since 1985, the Bisexual Resource Center has been committed to providing support to the bisexual community and raising public awareness about bisexuality and bisexual people.

Gay and Lesbian Alliance against Defamation (GLAAD)
www.glaad.org

This organization works with news media, entertainment media, social media, and cultural institutions to help shape the public's view of LGBTQIA+ people.

Gay, Lesbian, and Straight Education Network (GLSEN)
www.glsen.org
GLSEN works to ensure that LGBTQIA+ students can learn and grow in a school environment free from bullying and harassment. It was founded in 1990, by a group of teachers. The site contains loads of information and references to help with various school-related issues.

Advocate Magazine Online
www.advocate.com
This is a reliable source of gay, lesbian, bisexual, transgender, and queer news, including politics, commentary, arts, and entertainment, for more than fifty years.

Asexual Visibility and Education Network
www.asexuality.org
This site calls itself the world's largest online asexual community. It also contains a vast archive of resources on asexuality.

Lambda Legal
www.lambdalegal.org
Lambda Legal is a national organization committed to achieving full recognition of the civil rights of lesbians, gay men, bisexuals, transgender people, and everyone living with HIV through litigation, education, and public-policy work.

FOR THE ENTIRE FAMILY

For anyone who loves and supports you, or maybe doesn't support you yet because they don't understand LGBTQIA+ issues, these resources can help.

Parents and Friends of Lesbians and Gays (PFLAG)
www.pflag.org
The first and largest organization for LGBTQIA+ people and their parents, families, and allies, PFLAG was founded in 1973, as the simple act of a mother publicly supporting her gay son. If your parents or loved ones are asking questions and trying to understand or find a way to support you, this organization's website is a good place to send them.

Family Acceptance Project
familyproject.sfsu.edu
The Family Acceptance Project is a research, intervention, education, and policy initiative working to prevent the health and mental health risks for LGBTQIA+ children and youth, including suicide, homelessness, and HIV, in the context of their families, cultures, and faith communities.

HealthyChildren.Org (from the American Academy of Pediatrics)
www.healthychildren.org/English/ages-stages/teen/dating-sex/Pages/
Gay-Lesbian-and-Bisexual-Teens-Facts-for-Teens-and-Their-Parents.aspx
This is an excellent place to send your parents or guardians if they have questions or are struggling with understanding your sexual orientation, with lots of useful, factual information about gay people and advice for parents and caregivers.

American Psychological Association
www.apa.org/helpcenter/sexual-orientation
This site provides accurate information on sexual orientation and gender identity to share with your family and other loved ones.

Answer: Sex Ed, Honestly
answer.rutgers.edu/page/training
This sex education resource is aimed at providing high-quality training to teachers and other youth-serving professionals. Included are

online workshops, webinars, and other resources about LGBTQIA+ inclusive sex education and more.

Fortunate Families
www.fortunatefamilies.com
This supportive resource and networking ministry is for Catholic parents of LGBTQIA+ children.

True Colors United
truecolorsunited.org
True Colors United implements innovative solutions to youth homelessness that focus on the unique experiences of LGBTQIA+ young people.

FROM YOUR PEERS

If you are looking for stories and advice from other LGBTQIA+ youth and adults who can relate to your concerns and empathize with your issues, check out these references. You can also search YouTube and Google for "videos about coming out." You'll be inspired, uplifted, and maybe even get a little teary. Get ready for the feels.

I'm from Driftwood
www.imfromdriftwood.com
This is a collection of online videos described as "true stories from gay people all over."

Q Chat Space
www.qchatspace.org
Q Chat Space is a digital LGBTQIA+ center where teens can join live-chat, professionally facilitated online support groups.

It Gets Better Project
itgetsbetter.org

The It Gets Better Project inspires people throughout the world to share their stories and remind the next generation of LGBTQIA+ youth that there is hope and it will get better.

CenterLink: LGBT Centers
www.lgbtcenters.org
The motto of CenterLink is "developing strong LGBT centers and creating healthy LGBT communities." The organization's member directory can be used to find a center in your area.

QueerBFF
QueerBFF is a networking app that helps you find platonic friendships with other LGBTQIA+ people and connect with the LGBTQIA+ community wherever you are. You can find it on the Apple Store or Google Store online.

FAITH RESOURCES

If your faith is a big part of your identity and being ostracized from your church community is a real fear (or has already become a reality), other faith communities will welcome and embrace you.

Gay Buddhist Fellowship
www.gaybuddhist.org
The Gay Buddhist Fellowship is an organization for LGBTQIA+ Buddhists and their allies, families, and friends.

Axios
www.axios.org
This is an organization for Eastern Orthodox, Byzantine Rite, and Eastern Catholic LGBTQIA+ Christians.

Equally Blessed
www.equally-blessed.org

Equally Blessed is an organization of Catholics committed to full equality for LGBTQIA+ people in the church and civil society.

Affirmation LGBTQ Mormons, Families, and Friends
www.affirmation.org
This organization supports LGBTQIA+ and same-sex-attracted Mormons and their families, friends, and church leaders.

Affirmation
www.umaffirm.org
This organization challenges the United Methodist Church to be inclusive and radically speaks out against injustice for LGBTQIA+ people throughout the world.

Association of Welcoming and Affirming Baptists
www.awab.org
The Association of Welcoming and Affirming Baptists is an organization working to build the Welcoming and Affirming movement within the Baptist traditions.

Believe Out Loud
www.believeoutloud.com
This online network empowers Christians to work for LGBTQIA+ equality.

Brethren Mennonite Council for LGBTQ Interest
www.bmclgbt.org
This organization is creating an inclusive church and caring for the Mennonite and Brethren LGBTQ/allied community.

Covenant Network of Presbyterians
www.covnetpres.org
The Covenant Network of Presbyterians is a national group of Presbyterian clergy and lay leaders working toward a fully inclusive church.

Emergence International
www.emergence-international.org
    Emergence International is a community of Christian Scientists, their families, and friends providing spiritual and educational support for LGBTQIA+ people.

The Fellowship
www.radicallyinclusive.com
    This coalition of Christian churches is committed to radical inclusive ministry.

Muslim Alliance for Sexual and Gender Diversity
www.muslimalliance.org
    This organization is working to support, empower, and connect LGBTQIA+ Muslims.

Muslims for Progressive Voices
www.mpvusa.org
    This inclusive community is rooted in the traditional Qur'anic ideals of human dignity and social justice.

Institute for Judaism and Sexuality
www.huc.edu/ijso
    This organization is working toward a complete inclusion and welcoming of LGBTQIA+ Jews in communities and congregations.

Keshet
www.keshetonline.org
    This organization is working for the full equality and inclusion of LGBTQIA+ Jews in Jewish life.

Nehirim
www.nehirim.org
    Nehirim is a national community of LGBTQIA+ Jews, families, and allies committed to a more just and inclusive world.

The Gay and Lesbian Vaishnava Association, Inc.
www.galva108.org
    This religious organization offers positive information and support to LGBTQIA+ Vaishnavas and Hindus, as well as their allies, families, and friends.

Interweave
www.uua.org/lgbtq
    This is an organization working for LGBTQIA+ Unitarian Universalists and their allies, families, and friends.

LGBTQ Humanist Council
www.lgbthumanists.org
    The LGBTQ Humanist Council is a forum for LGBTQIA+ Humanists and allies to come together, build community, and work together to achieve full social and civil equality.

GLAAD Religion, Faith, and Values Program
www.glaad.org/programs/faith
    This program of GLAAD is working to amplify the voices of LGBTQIA-affirming communities of faith and LGBTQIA+ people of faith.

HRC Foundation's Religion and Faith Program
www.hrc.org/religion
    This program of the HRC is working to shape a world where no one has to choose between who they are, who they love, and what they believe.

FOR MORE ABOUT SEX

For more information about sex as it pertains to queer people, check out the following helpful sites.

The Trevor Project's Sexual Health Resources
www.thetrevorproject.org/trvr_support_center/sexual-health/
     In addition to all the other great resources, the Trevor Project has some excellent resources for more information about sex.

It's Your Sex Life
www.itsyoursexlife.com
     This partnership between Planned Parenthood and MTV supports young people in making responsible decisions about sexual health.

Healthline's LGBTQIA Safe-Sex Guide
www.healthline.com/health/lgbtqia-safe-sex-guide
     Healthline's LGBTQIA Safe-Sex Guide is the ultimate LGBTQIA+ guide to safe sex. It answers all your questions in a considerate and accurate way.

LGBTQ+ Resource Center at the University of Wisconsin
uwm.edu/lgbtrc/support/relationships-and-sex/
     Sponsored and authored by the University of Wisconsin–Milwaukee, this website contains lots of resources and information on relationships and sex.

INDEX

ABOUT THE AUTHOR

Kezia Endsley is a writer and editor from Indianapolis, Indiana. In addition to editing technical publications and writing books for teens, she also enjoys running and participating in triathlons, traveling, reading, and spending time with her family and many pets. She has written more than fifteen books for the teen market, including many about finding your best career.

CPSIA information can be obtained
at www.ICGtesting.com
Printed in the USA
LVHW091311280321
682728LV00005B/1134